#8650.4   15

Dr. Joel R. Beeke
2115 Romence Ave., N.E.
Grand Rapids, MI 49503

HEALING
AND
HOLINESS

BT 732.5 .S86 1990 JRB
Storms, C. Samuel, 1951-
Healing and holiness

Disc____ __d
____

D1502619

Puritan Reformed
Theological Seminary
2965 Leonard Street NE
Grand Rapids. MI 49525

HEALING AND HOLINESS

A BIBLICAL RESPONSE TO THE FAITH-HEALING PHENOMENON

C. Samuel Storms

Presbyterian and Reformed Publishing Company
Phillipsburg, New Jersey

Copyright © 1990 by C. Samuel Storms

All rights reserved. No part of this book may be reproduced in any form or by any means, except for brief quotations for the purpose of review, comment, or scholarship, without written permission from the publisher, Presbyterian and Reformed Publishing Company, Box 817, Phillipsburg, New Jersey 08865.

Unless otherwise indicated Scripture quotations are from the New American Standard Bible, copyright by the Lockman Foundation, 1960, 1962, 1963, 1968, 1971, 1972, 1973, 1975, 1977.

Excerpts taken from *A Step Further* by Joni Eareckson and Steve Estes. Copyright 1978 by Joni Eareckson and Steve Estes. Used by permission of Zondervan Publishing House.

Manufactured in the United States of America.
Typesetting by Thoburn Press, Box 2459, Reston, Virginia 22090.

Library of Congress Cataloging-in-Publication Data

Storms, C. Samuel, 1951-
     Healing and Holiness / by C. Samuel Storms
          p.   cm.
     Includes bibliographical references.
     ISBN 0-87552-446-X
     1. Spiritual healing.   2. Health—Biblical teaching.
     3. Evangelists—United States—Controversial literature.
     4. Pentecostalism—United States—Controversial literature.
     I. Title.
     BT732.5.S86   1990
     243'.13—dc20   89-38115
                                                            CIP

96   95   94   93   92   91   90   5   4   3   2   1

IN MEMORY OF

JOHN WATERMAN SLEDGE
(1958-88)

"He will wipe every tear from their eyes.
There will be no more death or mourning
or crying or pain, for the old order of
things has passed away" (Rev. 21:4).

CONTENTS

FOREWORD

Not even the most zealous Christians attain perfect holiness and
perfect maturity in this life. We reach after perfection and move toward it, but none of us arrives at it. We gain wisdom, but none of
us becomes fully wise. Nor is our spiritual growth uniform; blind
spots and weak points mar us all till we die. So we should never be
surprised at wild swings of the church's pendulum of interest, nor
at doctrinal nosedives now and then by honored teachers. Nor
should we doubt the value of that form of fellowship between believers that we call controversy, in which one sieves another's arguments to see what strength they have, thus doing his best to keep
the church healthy and honest, and to safeguard saints against
making mistakes.

The question of physical healing by direct act of God has been
under debate among evangelical Protestants for the past century.
In this debate the healing of the body has regularly been isolated
from the healing of the person, as if the body-soul dualism of ancient and modern philosophies were true, and the biblical view of
man as a psycho-physical unity (an ensouled body, or an embodied
soul) were false, and as if God's will to change our character had
nothing to do, one way or the other, with his will regarding our
physical health. But man should not separate what God has joined!
On the basis of this separation, interest in bodily healing has
grown in recent years: partly because physical health and pain-free
living have become obsessions in our culture, partly because it is
thought (wrongly, I believe) that medically inexplicable healings
will commend the gospel in the modern West, and partly because a
number of bold instructors have appeared to assure us that through
their own prayers, or through prayer techniques that they will

teach us, supernatural cures will regularly be given. That, of course, sounds exciting; but what is exciting is not necessarily right-minded. It might be biblically groundless. Or it might be an unworthy, worldly interest. Or it might be both. There is need to look, to see.

That is what Sam Storms's book does. It impresses me as soundly biblical in its perspectives and pastorally wholesome in its thrust. Not everyone will love him for writing in these terms, but every-one will benefit from weighing his arguments. I commend *Healing and Holiness* most heartily.

J. I. Packer

1

THE HEALING PHENOMENON

A Personal History

My first experience with what has become known as "charismatic Christianity" came in the summer of 1970. I was living in Lake Tahoe, Nevada, while actively involved in an evangelistic project sponsored by a well-known para-church organization.

At one point during the summer I drove from Lake Tahoe to Berkeley, California, and spent some time with people from The Christian World Liberation Front. You have no way of knowing how much of a shock that was for me. I had been raised in a conservative Southern Baptist church in Oklahoma where the "Jesus freaks" of southern California were considered an embarrassment to the name of Christ. "Hippies" were "hippies," religious zeal notwithstanding. But I found their faith refreshing. Their nonconformist approach to Christianity and worship shook my spiritual foundations.

When I returned to Tahoe, several of us involved in the project attended a meeting at which Harald Bredesen, one of the early leaders of the charismatic movement, was scheduled to speak. It was there that I heard of a book by John Sherrill entitled *They Speak With Other Tongues*. Upon returning to Oklahoma at the end of the summer I obtained a copy of the book and read it with unbridled zeal. Speaking in tongues became an obsession with me.

I had never so much as heard of the experience prior to my summer in California. (From what I understand there are a lot of people who hear about things for the first time in California!) I was concerned that I might be missing out on a spiritual blessing essential to my Christian growth. I prayed earnestly that if the gift were real, God would give it to me. For several weeks I spent each night in a secluded

1

area near my fraternity house pleading with God for some indication of his will for me concerning this spiritual phenomenon.

Then it happened. Without warning I suddenly lost control of my speech, pouring forth words of uncertain sound and form. I distinctly remember a somewhat detached sensation—sitting back, as it were, and listening to what seemed to be linguistic nonsense. It was unlike anything I had ever experienced before. All the while I was thinking to myself, "Sam, you don't even know what you're saying. Is this really it? Are you actually speaking in tongues?" To be perfectly honest, although it was emotionally and spiritually exhilarating, I was frightened. I just didn't know what was happening. I even tried to stop but couldn't. After about 45 seconds, it ceased as suddenly as it had begun.

Much as I tried, I never again experienced anything remotely similar to what happened that night. I'm not even sure what actually occurred. All I can say with certainty is that I experienced an amazing emotional surge. Whether it was of God or self-induced is difficult to say. I don't deny that it was spiritually exhilarating, but I'm not able to affirm anything beyond that.

Not long thereafter a friend whom I had been discipling in a Bible study startled me with word that he had seen a man's leg lengthened. He wanted my opinion. I felt totally unqualified to pass judgment on such a phenomenon until I had examined Scripture or had opportunity to witness it myself. We then learned that the evangelist who had allegedly performed this miraculous cure was holding a series of meetings in the ballroom of a Holiday Inn in nearby Oklahoma City. Several of us piled into a car and drove to the meeting.

As a Southern Baptist I had been to dozens of revivals in my 20 years, but none of them compared with what I witnessed that evening in Oklahoma City. Though the ballroom was packed, we were fortunate (and bold) enough to find several vacant seats in the front row. There were lots of singing, clapping of hands, and other activities associated with charismatic worship, none of which seemed objectionable. Then the preaching began. The evangelist told of an experience he had had similar to that of the apostle Paul who, according to 2 Corinthians 12, had been translated into the third heaven, into paradise itself. The speaker claimed that he had been translated into the very presence of Jesus Christ, who proceeded to pour oil on his head and hands and to commission him to take this newly bestowed healing power to all nations. Given my religious background, his story sounded more like an episode of "The Twilight Zone" than a sermon! The remainder of the message was filled with stories of miraculous cures God had wrought through him—everything from terminal cancer to cold sores.

Then things really took off. The organist began playing softly as the evangelist called for people who desired healing to line up in front of him. Before long the organist had climbed a couple of octaves, lifting us (perhaps even manipulating us) out of our seats in an emotional tidal wave. Those who had come forward stood eagerly awaiting their turns to have hands laid upon their heads. The result in each case was the same. They were "slain in the Spirit," falling backwards to the floor, and were caught by an usher or assistant to the evangelist. Some who were "slain" lay writhing upon the floor for several minutes, while others stood up after only a few seconds.

I was both fascinated and a bit frightened by it all. One thing was certain: my interest in the phenomenon of "divine healing" was kindled and today is little short of a raging fire. That is why I have written this book. My purpose is to share with you what I have discovered through my study of Scripture on this subject and to assess the claims being made by those involved in healing ministries today. Before I do so, permit me to make a few relevant observations on how to examine the validity of divine healing fairly and objectively.

Biblical Sanctions Versus Biased Judgments

First, I put no stock in experience that is devoid of scriptural sanction. If the Bible says yes to divine healing today, our traditional biases against it must go. But if the Bible says no, our experiences must be judged accordingly. If we are not willing to subordinate our experiences, desires, expectations, and wishes to the standard of the inspired and infallible Word of God, there is little sense in going any further in this study. We simply must acknowledge that the Bible is the objective rule for validating all subjective experiences.

A second important consideration has to do with the way charismatics and noncharismatics think of each other.[1] Those convinced that God wants to heal people today just as he did in the first century often accuse others of being sub-Christian and of denying the "fullness" of the Spirit's ministry. People occasionally telephone our church and ask if we are "full gospel." When I insist that we are, and note also that we are noncharismatic, an argument usually follows, though that is not my intention. I do believe in the "fullness" of Holy Scripture and of the ministry of the Holy Spirit. After all, if other churches are "full gospel" does that mean the rest of us are "three-quarters gospel" or "half gospel" or perhaps even "empty gospel"? I certainly hope not! How "full" our gospel is and how "full" the ministry of the Spirit is in our church can only be determined by what the Bible defines as "fullness." If we believe all that Scripture teaches and seek to practice all that Scripture commands, then we are as "full" as the next church, regardless of what label we bear.

Some charismatic authors insist that noncharismatics "put God in a box" when they question the validity of alleged healings. Others argue that since healings were a vital part of Jesus' ministry, anyone who opposes them opposes him. Noncharismatics "explain away" the Bible, or so we are told by some, though, not all charismatics.

On the other side noncharismatics can be just as unfair. They often conclude that since charismatics are big on experience, they must be soft on theology. While emotional displays may often be shallow,[2] they do not necessarily invalidate divine healing for our day. Rather than view enthusiasm with immediate suspicion, noncharismatics could do with a bit more emotional fervor themselves. Christianity without emotion is unthinkable as well as dull. To know the doctrines of grace but not feel anything is inconceivable. Not that everyone must express his or her emotional response to the truth in the same way. But those who prefer a more traditional and formal approach to worship must not denounce others who are a bit more flexible and exhuberant in the way they praise God. Whether we are discussing modes of worship or divine healing, the only relevant consideration is and always will be, "What does the Scripture say?"

Perhaps the greatest barrier to an objective assessment of divine healing is the tendency among noncharismatics to judge the theological accuracy of the majority on the basis of the aberrations of a minority. Too often we hear of something bizarre and proceed to paint the entire charismatic movement with the brush of our disdain. For example, consider this account by Kenneth Hagin concerning his "tour of hell."

> I went down, down, down, until the lights of the earth faded away. . . . The further down I went, the hotter it was and the more stifling it became. . . . I sensed that one more foot, one more step, one more yard, and I would be forever gone and could not come out of that horrible place. . . . I began to ascend until I came to the top of the pit and saw the light of the earth. I came back into it through the door, with the exception that my spirit needed no doors. I slipped back into my body as a man slips into his trousers in the morning, the same way in which I had gone out—through my mouth.[3]

Or what about Norvel Hayes who gives this description of what happened after he touched a lady who was both crippled and blind.

> When I did [touch her], the Holy Spirit's power picked her body up out of the wheelchair, and floated her through the air. . . . The Holy Spirit whirled her right through the air, and when she hit the floor everything about her was normal: her hand, her feet, her eyes. (Today she walks in high heels.)[4]

Hayes also relates an experience he had while in Columbus, Ohio. The Lord, says Hayes,

> came right through the wall of my motel room! I had been kneeling beside the bed praying, and it scared me so bad that some of my hair fell out and the meat on my body trembled. I jumped up on the bed and dug my heels into the bedspread. I backed up against the wall like a crayfish. . . . The Holy Ghost in my belly was jumping and tears were gushing out of

my eyes. Then I couldn't see. I thought the meat on my face was going to melt off my bones and go right on the floor. The Lord started talking to me in a voice. Now I'm not describing some sort of vision that I dreamed up. God Himself spoke to me *in a voice*![5]

William M. Branham, one of the founding fathers of the contemporary faith healing movement, claimed to have received a vision of an angel who told him that he would be able to detect diseases by vibrations in his left hand. He later claimed to have resurrected a fish (!) which had been killed by a friend.[6] And we all know of Oral Roberts's claim to have seen a nine-hundred-foot Jesus, as well as his appeal for $8 million based on God's threat to kill him if his followers failed to respond by the appointed date.

Whatever we may think of these claims, and they are more common than most people are aware, we simply may not prejudge the question of divine healing based upon them. Outlandish claims and extreme behavior notwithstanding, the concept of healing deserves to be heard and evaluated on its own *biblical* merits. Even if the above-mentioned examples are *not* the minority but represent mainstream charismatic Christianity, our responsibility to examine their claims objectively remains unchanged.

Reasons for Skepticism

Besides the bizarre methods described above there are, of course, other reasons why evangelical believers are cautious and skeptical of claims to miraculous divine healing. Some of these reasons are legitimate, whereas others are not. Not long ago the world-famous magician James Randi, in cooperation with the Committee for the Scientific Examination of Religion, uncovered what he alleged to be outright trickery and deceit on the part of a few TV evangelists. W. V. Grant, for example, claimed to possess divinely revealed information (called a "word of knowledge") concerning individuals in his audience, specifically their bodily ailments and diseases. After extensive examination of such claims Randi and his team of investigators concluded that Grant was using crib sheets and a mentalist's memory act. According to the humanist Paul Kurtz, editor of the magazine *Free Inquiry*, Grant "had obtained prior knowledge about the person who came to be healed: either from letters written to him or from information gleaned earlier in the evening by Grant or his confederates."[7]

Kurtz also claims to have "new and incontrovertible evidence" that Peter Popoff's hotline to heaven is actually a radio hookup from his wife backstage! "We have confirmed the fact," says Kurtz, "that Popoff—perhaps the most flamboyant of the TV evangelists—has a small receiver inserted in his ear. The so-called messages from God are really messages from Mrs. Popoff backstage. This cruel hoax is being perpetrated on helpless and innocent people who are waiting for divine deliverance."[8] I am not particularly pleased with having to rely on information supplied by a journal that is openly antithetical to the orthodox Christian faith. Nevertheless, if these charges are true, it is certainly understandable why noncharismatic Christians, as well as non-Christians, are less than ecstatic when they hear of "miraculous" healings and the like.

Also contributing to the skepticism of many is the subtle influence of Western materialism and secularism. Whether we are willing to admit it or not, the fact remains that we in the West are often unconsciously affected by the highly industrialized, technological, and scientific character of our society. People today generally take for granted that for every physical effect there must be a physical cause. Every phenomenon can be explained rationally and scientifically without appeal to a nonphysical or spiritually transcendent being such as God. This is clearly the operative philosophy throughout James Randi's earlier book, *Flim-Flam: Psychics, ESP, Unicorns, and Other Delusions* (Buffalo: Prometheus Books, 1982), in which he exposes the fraudulent claims, for example, of the psychic surgeons in the Philippines and other practitioners of alleged paranormal activities.

But no biblical Christian would ever knowingly doubt the reality of the supernatural or the power of God to produce physical effects by spiritual means. Christians wholeheartedly affirm their belief in the miracles recorded in Scripture, such as the virgin birth of Christ and his bodily resurrection from the dead. They wholeheartedly believe in divine providence over the world in general own lives in particular. "But even for orthodox believers," says John Wimber, "the effects of secularisation are far more subtle. While not creating outright rejection of the possibility of supernatural phenomena or the working of divine providence, especially events surrounding the first-century life of Christ, secularism *inclines* Christians to question modern reports of the supernatural."[9]

Although I have a few reservations concerning Wimber's approach to divine healing, on this point I must concur. Mainstream evangelicals are often wary of claims about the supernatural for other than biblical reasons, whether they are aware of those reasons or not. We therefore must consciously articulate our perspective on the world and God's relation to it if we are to investigate fairly the claims for divine healing in our day. On this point I heartily agree with the position taken by Lewis Smedes. He writes:

> We may begin by affirming that we view our world as a God-permeated cosmos. The God above all things is present with power in every dimension, material or mental, physical or spiritual, of our universe. The transcendent God is also the intangible energy behind all tangible energies, the cause of all natural causes. His Spirit is active, creating and preserving human life, replenishing its power to resist the negative forces of decay and disease and endlessly weaving the fabric of living cells. He gives life to the fragile flesh of his children. He moves every being toward its unique end. He provides all that creatures receive to nourish and sustain their lives; he is nature's secret healer, the mysterious power within nature to overcome its everpresent enemy, death. . . .

> We thus reject any world-picture in which God only occasionally invades the world via some interstices of nature or through some gaps unfilled by natural processes, to work an occasional miracle. We reject any script for the world in which God only now and then breaks through the hard crust of alien nature, overcomes its impersonal laws, and rescues isolated individuals from disease-bearing demons. We reject these views, not because they make too much of God's occasional demonstration of power, but because they make too little of God's constant presence and power.[10]

Smedes is led to this conclusion concerning miracles:

> In the biblical view, a miracle is a signal that God is, for a moment and for a special purpose, walking down paths he does not usually walk. A miracle is not a sign that a God who is usually absent is, for the moment, present. It is only a sign that God who is always present in creative power is working here and now in an unfamiliar style.[11]

Smedes reminds us that the author of miracles, which may be said to occur *in spite of* nature, is also the author of all that occurs *in* and *through* nature. God is as much the cause of gravity as he is the cause of the resurrection of Christ. The mistake many people make is in thinking that God acts only in the bizarre and unusual. The Bible says otherwise. Therefore if Christians in the Western world have unwittingly excluded God from the natural realm, believing that he is restricted to an exclusively spiritual sphere, they had better reassess their view of God.

Do I Believe in Miracles?

The answer to the question that you are undoubtedly asking is, Yes, I *do* believe in miraculous divine healing today. But note carefully my choice of words. Miraculous divine healing is *divine*. If someone is healed it is because *God* has chosen to do so, and not because of the power or promises of any human healer. But more important still, miraculous divine healing is *miraculous*. However else one may wish to define a "miracle," an essential element is that it is rare, not the rule. It is an exceptional and altogether unexpected act of God, not subject to human prediction or control.

A miracle is by definition improbable. "They would not be miracles," observes Colin Brown, "if they were not improbable."[12] When Oral Roberts regularly exhorts his audience, "Expect a miracle!" his words are a blatant contradiction. If an event is something you can with good reason *expect* will happen, it ceases to be miraculous. It becomes ordinary, predictable, and routine. The constant hankering for the miraculous and the spectacular was severely denounced by our Lord (Matt. 12:39; 16:4) as well as the apostle Paul

(1 Cor. 1:22). That sort of approach to Christian living in which one "expects" a miracle serves only to instill in people "the habit of not being moved unless they see a wonder. They want something bigger and better each time. They cease to wonder at the usual. If familiarity does not exactly breed contempt, it often breeds indifference."[13] The tragic consequence is that the beauty in nature itself is reduced to the bland and uninspiring.

It is this tendency on the part of some charismatics which J. I. Packer appropriately calls "super-supernaturalism"—affirming the supernatural in a way that exaggerates its discontinuity with the natural. Packer explains:

> Reacting against flat-tire versions of Christianity, which play down the supernatural and so do not expect to see God at work, the super-supernaturalist constantly expects miracles of all sorts—striking demonstrations of God's presence and power —and he is happiest when he thinks he sees God acting contrary to the nature of things, so confounding common sense. For God to proceed slowly and by natural means is to him a disappointment, almost a betrayal. But his undervaluing of the natural, regular, and ordinary shows him to be romantically immature and weak in his grasp of the realities of creation and providence as basic to God's work of grace.[14]

We should also be aware that many of those most vocal in the charismatic movement today are not merely affirming belief in miraculous divine healing. They are affirming belief in the virtual *certainty* of miraculous divine healing, if specified conditions are met. On their view it is the *absence* of healing that is the exception. The rule is that God wills to heal and shall heal. One may justifiably expect God to act today in precisely the same way he acted in the first century. If God did it then, he will do it now. If the required human conditions are fulfilled, God is under obligation to respond. It is this message so frequently proclaimed today that I find objectionable. I agree with David Hubbard that the one who suffers most from this approach to divine healing is God himself.

> Setting fixed terms which decide whether he performs healing or not nudges us across the border that separates providence

from magic and trespasses on God's right to be Lord. It pre-empts his authority to decide when and how to manifest his power. It makes our conformity to certain conditions rather than his sovereignty the ultimate ground of how he works. In the process, everyone loses. We find it hard to cling to God's love when healing does not take place, and God becomes servant of our needs and not Master of our destiny.[15]

What accounts for this modern obsession with healing? Undoubtedly we could cite numerous factors, but two immediately come to mind—one is social, and the other spiritual. On the one hand there is the over-all health craze in American society. New fangled diets, jogging, aerobics, health clubs, the threat of excessive salt and cholesterol in our food, the increase in heart disease, the AIDS epidemic, as well as rising medical costs, have all heightened our concern for good health.

But these phenomena alone are not sufficient to account for the beliefs and behavior of charismatic Christians. There is a decidedly spiritual explanation that must be noted. It is what J. I. Packer calls *eudaemonism*:

I use this word for the belief that God means us to spend our time in this fallen world feeling well and in a state of euphoria based on that fact. Charismatics might deprecate so stark a statement, but the regular and expected projection of euphoria from their platforms and pulpits, plus their standard theology of healing, show that the assumption is there, reflecting and intensifying the "now I am happy all the day, and you can be too" ethos of so much evangelical evangelism since D. L. Moody. Charismatics, picking up the healing emphasis of original restorationist Pentecostalism . . . regularly assume that physical disorder and discomfort are not ordinarily God's beneficent will for his children.[16]

When this is combined with other factors to be examined in the next several chapters, it is no wonder that the expectation of miraculous healing is so high, and the disappointment when it fails to occur is so devastating.

2

TWO CRUCIAL TEXTS:
HEBREWS 13:8 AND ISAIAH 53:4-5

The day was November 11, 1986. I was watching Pat Robertson's "700 Club" with special interest as an attractive young woman spoke of her miraculous healing. She had suffered from multiple sclerosis, which had left her partially paralyzed and totally blind. Although her condition was bleak she refused to accept it, insisting that her God was a great and good God and could heal her.

She then described for the TV audience a "vision" that came to her —something similar to a flashing neon sign in the sky, visible to no one but herself. The sign read, "This multiple sclerosis is a spirit." She immediately visited her church where the pastor "took authority" over the spirit, as a result of which she was instantly and wholly healed.

I do not know this woman's present condition, but if she is free from her affliction, I rejoice with her in giving all the glory to God.[1] But my immediate concern upon hearing her testimony was for the hundreds, perhaps thousands, of viewers sitting at home in their living rooms who likewise suffer from MS or diabetes or cancer, and experience no healing. They, no less than she, are filled with faith, hope, and confidence in a God whom they, no less than she, know to be both great and good. Yet they see no vision, hear no voice, and remain in their affliction.

How are they supposed to feel? I'm afraid that at the same time they rejoice with her they begin to doubt themselves. "What's the matter with me? Is my faith deficient? Have I committed some sin?" The result is that there is added to the burden of a physical disability the even more unbearable pain of emotional and spiritual guilt, along with feelings of inadequacy, inferiority, and abandonment.

I suppose this is what disturbs me the most about modern healing ministries. They publicize the occasional "miracle" and praise the faith of the one healed, but conveniently ignore the multitudes who continue to suffer. The testimony I want to hear is of the person who suffers from a debilitating, perhaps terminal, illness and is *not* healed, yet whose faith in God remains unshaken. It is the remarkable life Joni Eareckson Tada lives from a wheelchair that bolsters me in my faith more than any dozen miracles of healing. It is what countless other Christian men and women are enabled by divine grace to do, in spite of ongoing illness, disability, or frailty, that encourages and inspires my Christian walk with the Lord.

But why do those involved in healing ministries insist that what this woman with MS experienced is normative? They tell us that God is as willing to heal others as he was to heal her. To be healed is the divine rule; to remain unhealed, the human exception. On what basis do they make such an assertion? In this chapter I want us to examine two passages of Scripture that are foundational to the charismatic position on divine healing. Because they are quoted more often in support of miraculous healing than are any other biblical texts, it is crucial that we familiarize ourselves with what they say.

Hebrews 13:8 and the Immutability of God

Perhaps the most frequently cited text in healing ministries is Hebrews 13:8. There we read that "Jesus Christ is the same yesterday and today, yes and forever." One of the attributes of our great Triune God is that he does not change; he is immutable. Therefore, if he healed people yesterday, he must certainly be willing to heal people today. Whatever he willed in the past he must will in the present. If not, God is not immutable. "For healing to pass away," says Gloria Copeland, "then God would have to pass away."[2]

Like so much error, there is an element of truth in this argument. God *is* immutable. Jesus Christ *is* the same yesterday, today, and forever. Our great Triune God neither gains nor loses attributes. There is neither increase nor decrease in God, either quantitatively or qualitatively. He neither evolves nor devolves. God will never be wiser, more loving, more powerful, or holier than he ever has been. He doesn't get better or worse. He is infinitely and always the best![3]

All I am saying is that God's nature or character does not change. What he has been from eternity past he will be into eternity future. However, to say that because God's *nature* is immutable, he must *do* in every age what he does in one age is erroneous. The immutability of God's nature simply means that what he *is*, he will always be. But the *way* in which God manifests himself to men and women and deals with them undoubtedly varies. Of course, *how* God relates to us is always a reflection of *who* he is, but that does not mean that he must always relate to us in precisely the same way he related to people in Old Testament or even in New Testament times.

For example, before the Mosaic law was given, men were free to eat anything. With the coming of the law, however, God prohibited Israel from eating pork and other food items. Subsequent to the cross we are all again free to eat anything, provided it is received with thanksgiving (1 Tim. 4:1-5). Surely no one would accuse God of being mutable or fickle in regard to what he permits men to eat.

Or let's take an example dear to the hearts of most charismatics: speaking in tongues (the example of "baptism in the Holy Spirit" would work just as well). There is no indication in Scripture that the spiritual gift of tongues, or the interpretation of tongues, was in operation prior to Pentecost. If any pre-Pentecost manifestation of tongues can be identified, it would be an isolated and exceptional case. Does this mean we are justified in charging God with being changeable? After all, if he is the same yesterday, today, and forever, why did he *begin* to do something at Pentecost that he had determined not to do before? If, as charismatics insist, the gift of tongues is a blessing given to us by a loving God for our spiritual welfare, what becomes of those believers in Old Testament times who never even heard of the phenomenon? Did God not love them as much as he loves us? Is the God who dispensed tongues at Pentecost different from the one about whom we read in the Old Testament? Of course not! But if divine immutability means that God must always do in one age of redemptive history what he does in another, we are driven to the unhappy conclusion that God is not immutable after all.

To assert flatly that God must perform the same works in every age is both theologically naive and simplistic. It is the result of emotional zeal and exuberance unbounded by a careful consideration of biblical truth. It exposes a failure to distinguish between *who God is* and *what God does*. Though God's character, his nature, his essential attributes never change, what God *does* with men and women and *how* he relates to them varies from age to age. Whatever God does is always morally and spiritually compatible with who he is; he never acts contrary to his nature. But that doesn't mean God always has to do the same thing for every person in every age, unless of course he has obligated himself by an explicit promise. God did things for Israel as a theocratic nation that he does not and will not do for us today, and vice versa. This is not to say he couldn't have done for them what he does for us, or that he is unable to heal today as he healed in the first century. *It is a matter not of God's power but of his purpose.* Whether or not God is as willing to heal today as he did in the first century is another question, which we have yet to discuss. *If* he is willing, he is just as capable now as he was then because his *character* and *ability* are immutable. But we have to ask whether miraculous healing is his *purpose* and *will* for today, an issue we shall address at length later.

Isaiah 53:4-5 and Healing in the Atonement

The second key passage used by charismatics to defend their notion of divine healing is Isaiah 53:4-5, along with Matthew 8:17 and 1 Peter 2:24 where it is cited. The passage in Isaiah says, "Surely our griefs [lit., "sicknesses"] He Himself bore, and our sorrows [lit., "pains"] He carried; yet we ourselves esteemed Him stricken, smitten of God, and afflicted. But he was pierced through for our transgressions, He was crushed for our iniquities; the chastening for our well-being fell upon Him, and by His scourging we are healed."

Let's begin by noting what the charismatics say about this text. Listen to the interpretation of A. J. Gordon.

> The yoke of his cross by which he lifted our iniquities took hold also of our diseases; so that it is in some sense true that as

God "made him to be sin for us who knew no sin," so he made him to be sick for us who knew no sickness. He who entered into mysterious sympathy with our pain which is the fruit of sin, also put himself underneath our pain which is the penalty of sin. In other words the passage seems to teach that Christ endured vicariously our diseases as well as our iniquities. If now it be true that our Redeemer and substitute bore our sick-nesses, it would be natural to reason at once that he bore them that we might not bear them.[4]

Gloria Copeland agrees with Gordon. She writes:

Jesus bore your sicknesses and carried your diseases at the same time and in the same manner that He bore your sins. You are just as free from sickness and disease as you are free from sin. You should be as quick to refuse sickness and disease in your body as you are to refuse sin.[5]

Colin Urquhart, a British pastor, says it as explicitly as one possi-bly can.

When Jesus stood bearing the lashes from the Roman soldiers, all our physical pain and sicknesses were being heaped upon him. . . . It is as if one lash was for cancer, another for bone disease, another for heart disease, and so on. Everything that causes physical pain was laid on Jesus as the nails were driven into His hands and feet.[6]

Such statements are baffling. We are being told that "Christ bore our sicknesses in the very same way that He bore our sins."[7] Gordon says that just as God made Jesus to be *sin* for us he also "made him to be *sick* for us." Again, he writes that "Christ endured vicariously our diseases as well as our iniquities."

We all know what the apostle Paul meant when he wrote in 2 Corinthians 5:21 that God "made Him who knew no sin to be sin on our behalf." He was declaring that the guilt of our sins was im-puted to Christ and that it was because of that guilt that he was punished in our place. But what can it possibly mean to say God made him "to be sick" on our behalf? Kenneth Hagin, who is considered by many to be the father of the modern "faith" movement, says that God "made him [Jesus] sick with your diseases that you might be perfectly well in Christ."[8] But there is no guilt in disease or sickness. Having diabetes or a head cold is not sinful. The Bible tells us to pray "forgive us our trespasses" and urges us "to confess our sins," but nowhere does it say that we should pray "forgive us our arthritis" or "Lord, I confess that I have the flu." *Sickness is not sin.* The Bible never issues the command, "Thou shalt not commit cancer," or "Flee the flu!" Nevertheless, charismatic authors such as Hugh Jeter insist that Jesus "bore the penalty for our sins and sicknesses."[9] But if sickness is not a sin, how can it incur a penalty?

Of course, ultimately all sickness is a result of sin, in that Adam's fall introduced corruption and death into the human race. But that does not mean that every time we get sick it is because of some specific sin we have committed. It *does* mean that had *Adam* not sinned, there would be no sickness. Sickness is the *effect* of sin (just like tornadoes, weeds, and sadness). But that is altogether different from saying that sickness *is* sin. We do not repent for having kidney stones, nor do we come under conviction for catching the measles. I didn't rebuke my nine-year-old daughter for coming down with the chicken pox, and I certainly didn't ask my three-year-old to ask for forgiveness when she caught it from her older sister!

Jesus was not punished for our diseases. Rather, he endured the wrath of God that was provoked by our willful disobedience of the truth.

So what does it mean in Isaiah 53 when it says that he bore our sicknesses and carried our pains and that by his stripes we are healed? I believe we have in this passage an example of a figure of speech frequently found in Scripture and in everyday conversation. It is called a *metonomy.* Although that sounds technical, it is really quite simple. For example, we read in Luke 16:29, "But Abraham said, 'They have Moses and the Prophets; let them hear them.'" What is meant is that they have the Scriptures *written by* Moses and the prophets. Moses and the prophets themselves, obviously, have long since died. The author has put the *cause* (Moses and the prophets) in place of the *effect* (the Scriptures), and this is called a *metonomy of cause for effect.* Had the figure of speech not been used the passage would have been, "But Abraham said, 'They have the Old Testament Scriptures [of which Moses and the prophets are the cause or authors]; let them hear them.'"

In 1 Peter 2:24 the apostle writes, "And He Himself bore our sins in His body on the cross." This is another example of metonomy where the cause (our sin) is put in place of the effect (penal judgment). Christ "bore our sins" in the sense that he bore the wrath of God of which our sins were the cause. We use this figure of speech all the time without ever knowing it. Have you ever said to someone, "Don't give me any of your lip!"? What you really meant was, "Don't use your lip(s) (or mouth) to give me any backtalk." Dozens of other examples from both Scripture and everyday speech could be cited (see especially Col. 3:5; 1 Thess. 5:19).

Then there is the flip side, as it were, in which the effect is put in place of the cause. After having seen the baby Jesus, Simeon declared, "For my eyes have seen Thy salvation" (Luke 2:30). That is, in seeing the cause of salvation (Jesus), Simeon had seen the effect (salvation). Or again, Jesus said to Martha, "I am the resurrection and the life" (John 11:25). The effects (resurrection and life) are put in place of the cause (Jesus' work and ministry).

In the case of Isaiah 53 we have an example of this latter form of metonomy in which the effect is put for the cause. Sin is the ultimate cause of which illness is one among many effects. Jesus bore our sicknesses in the sense that he was punished for the sin that causes sickness. He carried our pains, not in the sense of personally experiencing stomach viruses and ulcers and earaches and gallstones as he hung on Calvary's tree, but by enduring the wrath of God against that willful human wickedness which is ultimately the reason there are such things as pain and infirmity. By his death at his *first* coming he has laid the foundation for the ultimate overthrow and annihilation of all physical disease, which will occur with the resurrection of the body at his *second* coming. Thus it is theological nonsense to say Jesus bore our sicknesses in the same way he bore our sins. Rather, he paid the price of the latter (sin) in order that one day, when he returns to glorify his people, he may wholly do away with the former (sickness).

May we conclude that there is healing in the atonement? Of course! Were it not for Jesus making atonement for sin, we would have no hope of healing in any form, either now or later. The redemptive suffering of Jesus at Calvary is the foundation and source of *every* blessing, whether spiritual or physical. To ask Is there healing in the atonement? is like asking Is there forgiveness of sins in the atonement? or Is there fellowship with God in the atonement? There is even a sense in which we may say that the Holy Spirit is in the atonement! We are told in John 14:16-17, 26; 15:26; and especially 16:7-15 that the Holy Spirit's present ministry is a result of the death, resurrection, and exaltation of Jesus.

Everything we Christians receive from God finds it ultimate source in what Christ did for us on the cross. Therefore, the question is not *whether* our bodies receive healing because of the atonement of Christ, but *when*. We are forgiven of our sins *now* because of Christ's atoning death, but we await the consummation of our deliverance from the presence of sin when Christ returns. We experience fellowship with God *now* because of Christ's atoning death, but we await the consummation of that blessed relationship when Christ returns. We profit immensely *now* from the Spirit's work in our hearts, but who would dare suggest that what the Holy Spirit is doing in this age is all that he will ever do? There is a glorious harvest reserved in heaven for us of which the present ministry of the Holy Spirit is merely the first fruits!

In other words, it is a serious mistake for us to think that every blessing Christ secured through his redemptive suffering will be ours *now* in its consummate form. All such blessings shall indeed be ours; let there be no mistake about that. But let us not expect, far less demand, that we *now* experience fully those blessings which God has clearly reserved for heaven in the age to come.

Life for the believer in this present age is a life of tension between the "already" and the "not yet." We already have so very, very much. But we have not yet experienced it all. There is much yet to come. One of the "not yet's" in Christian experience is the redemption and glorification of the body. "For our citizenship is in heaven," says Paul, "from which also we eagerly wait for a Savior, the Lord Jesus Christ; who will transform the body of our humble state into conformity with the body of His glory, by the exertion of the power that He has even to subject all things to Himself" (Phil.

3:20-21). Paul tells us in Romans 8:18-25 that the consummation of our adoption as God's children, which he defines as the redemption of our *bodies*, is something we eagerly and anxiously await; it is a *future* experience for which we in the present "groan" (Rom. 8:23) in holy expectation. To insist that this physical blessing is future is not to detract from the efficacy or value of Christ's atoning work. It is simply to recognize, as Scripture does, that God's timing is often different from ours.

But what about Matthew 8:16-17? We are told that Jesus "healed all who were ill in order that what was spoken through Isaiah the prophet might be fulfilled, saying, 'He Himself took our infirmities, and carried away our diseases.'" The charismatic would have us believe that these healings performed by Jesus are in the atonement. Well of course they are. But it does not necessarily follow that where there is atonement there is always an immediate healing. This passage in Matthew only proves what I am sure all Christians affirm, namely, that whatever healing *does* occur comes as a result of Christ's redemptive work. But it does *not* mean that healing will *always* occur *now* as a result of that work.

In the case of 1 Peter 2:24 we have something different. Frequently in Scripture the sinful condition of the soul is portrayed as analogous to a body suffering from various wounds. Forgiveness and restoration are therefore described in terms of a bodily healing. For example, consider this description of the sinful condition of the nation Israel.

> Where will you be stricken again, as you continue in your rebellion? The whole head is sick, and the whole heart is faint. From the sole of the foot even to the head there is nothing sound in it, only bruises, welts, and raw wounds, not pressed out or bandaged, nor softened with oil (Isa. 1:5-6).

We find something similar in Isaiah 30:26 where the Lord "binds up the fracture of His people and heals the bruise He has inflicted." Through Jeremiah the Lord says to captive Israel:

> Your wound is incurable and your injury is serious. There is no one to plead your cause; no healing for your sore, no re-

covery for you. All your lovers have forgotten you, they do not seek you; for I have wounded you with the wound of an enemy, with the punishment of a cruel one, because your iniquity is great and your sins are numerous. Why do you cry out over your injury? Your pain is incurable. Because your iniquity is great and your sins are numerous, I have done these things to you. . . . For I will restore you to health and I will heal you of your wounds (Jer. 30:12-17).

Much of the same thing may also be found in Jeremiah 8:22; 2 Chronicles 7:14; and Matthew 13:15, just to mention a few passages.

This is what I believe we have in 1 Peter 2:24. The apostle portrays us in our sin as if we were a wounded body in need of physical healing. By his atoning death the Great Physician has truly "healed" our hearts. We were continually straying like sheep, but by the redemptive grace of Jesus we have been enabled to return to the shepherd and guardian of our souls (1 Pet. 2:25). Thus the context of 1 Peter 2:24 clearly tells us that it is spiritual "healing" from the disease of sin, not physical restoration of the body, that the apostle has in mind.

All Christians, whatever may be their opinion of the charismatic movement, should rejoice in the truth of Isaiah 53. Let us continually give thanks that there is bodily healing for us in the atonement of Jesus Christ. Let us forever acknowledge that whatever healing and health we experience now is a blessing that flows from Calvary's tree. But let us also remember that there are certain blessings that God intends to bestow in their consummate fullness only when the Lord Jesus returns. Until then we weep, suffer, and die. On that glorious day when the Savior appears, *then* shall come to pass the words of Revelation 21:3-4, "And I heard a loud voice from the throne, saying, 'Behold, the tabernacle of God is among men, and He shall dwell among them, and they shall be His people, and God Himself shall be among them, and He shall wipe away every tear from their eyes; and there shall no longer be any death; there shall no longer be any mourning, or crying, or pain; the first things have passed away.' "

3

HEALING AND HAPPINESS

I have often heard it said, "God wants everyone to be healed, because God wants everyone to be happy." The idea is that since God is good and wants the best for us, he will alleviate whatever diminishes our joy. If he doesn't, there must be a flaw in God's character. This argument is frequently expressed in terms of God's love for us. Francis MacNutt puts it this way:

> If we truly believe that God is love, then it should be easy to believe that healing is an ordinary, not an extraordinary sign of his compassion. Any other attitude toward healing robs the gospel of the reality of God's revelation of himself as a loving father.[1]

In another place MacNutt is even more explicit.

> When we say God sends sickness or asks us to endure it, we are creating for many people an image of God they must eventually reject. What human mother or father would choose cancer for their daughter in order to tame her pride; yet, this is the kind of punishment we portray God as putting upon his people.[2]

Such reasoning churns up our emotions and sounds persuasive on the surface. But I am convinced that it is both superficial and spurious. Let me explain why.

Joy Not Conditioned on Good Health

Those who follow MacNutt's reasoning make it sound as if they and their God are *for* human happiness whereas we and our God are *against* it. Nothing could be further from the truth. Of course

God wants his children to be happy. The only alternative to this is to say God wants us to be sad, which is ridiculous. "Rejoice always" (1 Thess. 5:16) is God's word to us through Paul. "Rejoice in the Lord always; again I will say, rejoice!" (Phil. 4:4). Well, then, if God really wants us to be happy, surely he must also want us to be healed, right? Not necessarily. Undoubtedly there *are* times when God wants to heal, and when he wants to he will, for which we should rejoice and give thanks. But the problem here is that most faith healers have a misguided and unscriptural notion of what constitutes "happiness."

In the New Testament "happiness" or "joy" does not necessarily mean the absence of physical pain or external adversity. Happiness is a delight in Jesus Christ that transcends earthly, outward circumstances. It is an inner contentment, a sense of well-being, which remains unaffected and unperturbed by worldly turmoil and bodily pain. When Paul wrote to the Philippian Christians from prison, notwithstanding the deprivation and bodily abuse he suffered, he called on them to make his *joy* complete "by being of the same mind, maintaining the same love, united in spirit, intent on one purpose" (Phil. 2:2). Later in the same epistle he told them: "I have learned to be content in whatever circumstances I am. I know how to get along with humble means, and I also know how to live in prosperity; in any and every circumstance I have learned the secret of being filled and going hungry, both of having abundance and suffering need. I can do all things [specifically, I can be content and happy regardless of the circumstances] through Him who strengthens me."

Christian happiness or joy is not like the mercury in a thermometer, rising and falling with the heat of the day. It is a constant, ever-deepening sense of delight in Christ. Paul was no less happy when he hurt, because the source of his joy was not physical pleasure, which may come and go, but Jesus Christ who is ever and always the same. If you cannot be happy unless you are healthy there is something woefully deficient in your understanding of God and his grace. The believer's joy is in the glory of God, not just his favorable providence. Not that the believer should be ungrateful for good health or want discomfort. But true spiritual happiness can exist, thrive, and deepen *aside from* physical health and external prosperity. If God should bless you with health and wealth, rejoice and give thanks. If not, rejoice nonetheless!

Holiness More Important Than Happiness

Another thing we must keep in mind is that whereas our happiness is certainly important to God, our holiness is even more important. In a later chapter I'll discuss the purposes of God in our suffering. For now I only want to remind you that sometimes the best, and perhaps the only, way to make us holy in this life is to make us hurt. Paul discovered this and wrote of it in 2 Corinthians 12:7-10 (see chapter 9). Unfortunately Francis MacNutt caricatures God in this view as a heartless parent who inflicts cancer on a child to tame his pride. But we must be very careful not to judge what God does based on what we do. We are not the measure or standard by which the morality and wisdom of God's actions are determined. The omniscient God is infinitely wise and knows our needs far better than we know our earthly children. He is able to see the ultimate spiritual profit he can bring out of our afflictions when we cannot (Rom. 8:28).

As the father of two daughters I must confess that on occasion I do deliberately diminish their immediate happiness and I do inflict bodily pain to curb their sin. It is called spanking. Whether or not God uses cancer to tame our pride is questionable, in that he always tailors the chastisement to fit the sin. But if our holiness can come only at the expense of our pleasure, comfort, or health, and I am convinced that sometimes it must, then we should be prepared to be humbled under the mighty hand of a loving Father. Perhaps part of the problem is our failure to realize that worse than any bodily disease is sin. Pride is a spiritual cancer that damages the soul far worse than any physical cancer ravages the body.

Genuine Christian love does not always manifest itself in providing immediate and total relief, even if that were possible. God often uses short-term, earthly grief to achieve eternal, heavenly glory. True love corrects and chastises (Heb. 12:4-11) no less than it comforts and consoles. Thus Paul can write:

Therefore we do not lose heart, but though our outer man is decaying, yet our inner man is being renewed day by day. For momentary, light affliction is producing for us an eternal weight of glory far beyond all comparison, while we look not at the things which are seen, but at the things which are not seen; for the things which are seen are temporal, but the things which are not seen are eternal (2 Cor. 4:16-18).

Kenneth Hagin takes up MacNutt's point, but with even greater vehemence.

If you had children, would it be your will that your children be sick and afflicted? Certainly not! Would it be your will that they go through life poverty stricken and begging? No, no, no![3]

In the first place, what *I* will or want is not relevant. What *God* wills and wants *is*. And the fact remains that no matter how much I think I may know what is best for my children, God knows infinitely more. Therefore, the answer to Hagin's first question is no, I don't enjoy seeing my children ill and in pain. And I will take every opportunity to alleviate their suffering. That is because I do not have divine insight into God's purpose for permitting them to be afflicted. But if God should providentially overrule my efforts to insure their health, in his concern for their even greater need for holiness, then I humbly submit to his will. Furthermore, I do *not* want my children to be *either* wealthy *or* poverty stricken. My prayer for them is the prayer of Proverbs 30:7-9: "Two things I asked of Thee, do not refuse me before I die; keep deception and lies far from me, give me neither poverty nor riches; feed me with the food that is my portion, lest I be full and deny Thee and say, 'Who is the Lord?' Or lest I be in want and steal, and profane the name of my God."

And yet, if God should choose to make my children wealthy, I pray that they would be thankful and wise in the use of their wealth, and that God might protect them from the temptations it brings. And if God should choose to make them poor, I pray that they would realize their treasure is in heaven, and that the only wealth truly worth having is the wealth that lasts: eternal life in Christ Jesus. We are not to seek poverty nor squander the material blessings we receive. But if God providentially overrules, let us never forget the example of the people described in Hebrews 11:36-40:

> Women received back their dead by resurrection; and others were tortured, not accepting their release, in order that they might obtain a better resurrection; and others experienced mockings and scourgings, yes, also chains and imprisonment. They were stoned, they were sawn in two, they were tempted, they were put to death with the sword; they went about in sheepskins, in goatskins, being destitute, afflicted, ill-treated (men of whom the world was not worthy), wandering in deserts and mountains and caves and holes in the ground. And all these, having gained approval through their faith, did not receive what was promised, because God had provided something better for us, so that apart from us they should not be made perfect.

What went wrong? Did these people suffer because they lacked faith? Certainly not. It is because of their faith that they were praised and through their faith that they gained approval. Were these people destitute because God did not love them? Certainly not. The fact is, nothing went wrong. The kind of life they lived is not unusual for those who love God and are called according to his purpose. We err when we conclude that such people are not worthy to live in this world. God looks on them and concludes that the world is not worthy to have them!

Finally, the assertion "God wills all to be healed because he wills all to be happy," if true, creates more problems than it solves. It assumes that because God is love, he must not and will not tolerate anything we perceive as damaging to ourselves. If that is true, why single out physical illness? If the principle is "God is willing to do away with whatever makes us unhappy," how do we explain other hardships in our lives, such as natural disasters, technical and mechanical breakdowns, decay, and death? Few things cause more emotional pain, heartache, and sadness than the death of a spouse. But we know that death, like so many other things that diminish our joy, will be abolished only at the second coming of the Savior.

My point is that this world, *your personal world*, is full of experiences that hurt and sadden you—including physical illnesses. God does not exempt his children from illness or disease any more than he exempts the faithful from tornadoes, shipwreck, car failure, aging, or physical death. We do not, or at least should not, accuse God of cruelty or heartlessness for declining to remove such adversities *right now*. Remove them he will! But not necessarily now. When Jesus returns, the curse upon the natural realm will be lifted, and we will see the end both to sin and to its consequences, not the least of which is bodily disease. The ultimate remedy for all ills —be they sins themselves or merely the effects of living in a fallen world—is the application of the redemptive work of Christ, the consummation of which will come only when he does. Even so, come Lord Jesus!

4

HEALING, FAITH, AND THE WILL OF GOD

Does God Always Desire to Heal?

As we noted in the preceding chapter, many charismatics actively involved in healing ministry believe that it is always God's will to heal. It is not enough for us to believe that God is *able* or has the power to heal us. We must also believe that he *wants* to do so. Anyone who wishes to be healed must have absolute certainty that that is God's purpose. One must rid his or her mind of all doubt and apprehension concerning God's desire to restore health. If God does not heal, it isn't because he is unwilling. It can only be due to a failure in our faith.

Lest you think I have overstated this position, let me cite a few examples. F. F. Bosworth, born in 1877, was one of the founding fathers of the modern healing revival. He once wrote that "it is impossible to have real faith for healing as long as there is the slightest doubt as to its being God's will."[1] Gloria Copeland unabashedly declares that "you must know that it is God's will to heal you. Until this fact is settled in your mind and spirit, you cannot approach healing without being double minded and wavering."[2] Again, she insists that "believing in healing is not enough. You must *know* that it is God's will for *you* to be healed."[3]

Colin Urquhart contends that "when you come tentatively with an 'if,' the first thing He [God] wants to do is to remove the 'if' from your thinking."[4] The proper attitude for a Christian is not "if God wills to heal me" but "*since* God wills to heal me." Therefore, to preface or conclude one's prayer for healing with the words "if it be Thy will" is destructive of true faith. " 'If it be Thy will,' " says Copeland, "is unbelief when praying for healing. There is no faith in that kind of praying. It is the opposite of faith."[5] When you look to the Lord for healing, "you should know that it is God's will to heal you *before* you ever pray."[6] Urquhart says that "if it be Thy will" is a "faith killing statement."[7]

What we are being told is that, far from an expression of humility and submission to God's sovereign purpose, "if it be Thy will" is a cop-out. It is tacked on to the end of a prayer to protect the Christian from the disillusionment that comes when he does not get what he prays for. The proviso "if it be Thy will" weakens our confidence in prayer and provides us with a psychological escape-hatch in the event that God says no. It is not good enough to say, "I believe God *can* heal me and I *hope* he will." One must be able to say, "I believe God *wants* to heal me and I *know* he will." To pray in any other way is to insult God by refusing to take him at his word.

Faith or Presumption?

Why do charismatics speak with such robust confidence concerning God's will? On what basis do they assert so boldly that they *know* God's will even before they pray? Several reasons for their assurance have already been discussed. They argue from Hebrews 13:8 that since God was willing to heal in the first century, he must be willing to heal in the twentieth century – God is always the same. And, they appeal to Isaiah 53 and insist that God must always be willing to heal because healing is in the atonement. After all, Jesus died to remove our sicknesses as well as our sins. They also believe God must be willing to heal because God is good, is loving, and wants nothing but happiness for his children. I responded to these arguments in chapters 2 and 3. Of course there are other reasons why charismatics are convinced God is not only able but also willing to heal today, which I will address in subsequent chapters.

Then, of course, there is the opposite side of the coin. Some charismatics turn the tables and suggest that if a believer is persuaded that it *is* God's will for him to be sick, it is *sinful* to pray for healing or to seek the help of a physician. Such confusion flows from the assumption that we can always know God's will for our health and healing. Consider, for example, the view of Gloria

Copeland. She says that if you believe God intends for you to be sick, "you need to quit taking your medicine. If it is God's will for you to be sick then to take medicine would be to fight against the will of God. If you really believe that, just roll up in a ball and die as quickly as you can."[8] Colin Urquhart says much the same thing.

> If God wants them [believers] to be sick and desires to be glorified in their illness, they should not seek any remedy or relief through prayer or the medical profession; that would make doctors active agents against God's will. To seek help would be to go against what they claim to be God's purpose. To be consistent they should suffer their pain willingly, glad to be at one with what they claim to be God's will.[9]

Now notice carefully the basis upon which both Copeland and Urquhart make these assertions. Both allude to an assumption that a Christian can *know* or at least have some degree of assurance that God wants him to be ill. Copeland writes, "If it is God's will for you to be sick . . ." Urquhart likewise writes, "If God wants them to be sick . . ." And again, he says that illness is "what they claim to be God's will." But the noncharismatic position does *not* suggest we can be certain that ill health is God's will for us. Aside from what Scripture explicitly asserts, we cannot be sure what God's will is in any particular situation.[10]

What we do know with certainty is that illness *may* be God's will for our lives. It is definitely within the realm of possibility that God permits us to be afflicted, as I hope to demonstrate in subsequent chapters. But that "maybe," that possibility, is never to be a deterrent to prayer for healing. If we were only to pray for things we knew were certainly God's will, we would rarely pray at all. Apart from what the Bible tells us, the future is unknown to us. What God may or may not will to accomplish is, to put it bluntly, none of our business. Our business is to act and pray responsibly on the basis of what is revealed in the Bible.

We have no biblical warrant for refusing to act responsibly based on what we speculate may or may not be God's sovereign will. The Bible endorses prayer at *all* times and instructs us to be wise, which would certainly apply to the use of modern medical science. If illness *is* God's will (it may or may not be), our prayers for health and the medicine we take will not avail. But our guesses about *whether* illness is God's will cannot be made the basis on which we respond to explicit biblical exhortations.

We should also remember that complete healing and health may be God's *ultimate*, long-range will for us, but not his immediate will. It may be that after God has fulfilled his purpose for our present suffering, he will restore us to physical wholeness through our persistent prayers and medical help. But since we can never *know* with certainty the mind of God *in this regard*, we are responsible to heed and to obey what we do know with certainty—what God has said in his Word. Thus we are always to avail ourselves of every medical aid to counteract a disease, while praying that, if it is God's will, he would heal us. If it is not his will, he will providentially overrule our efforts. But our efforts should never be considered resistance to God's will. He certainly does not look upon them in that light. Indeed, how can they be interpreted as fighting against God's purpose when we do not know what that purpose is?

If there is no biblical basis for asserting that God is always willing to heal, then what charismatics call "faith" comes perilously close to presumption. When the Bible speaks of faith, it means an attitude of humility and self-renunciation. Faith says, "Lord, I am nothing and you are everything; I entrust myself to your care, regardless of the outcome." Faith isn't a weapon by which we demand things from God; it is the way in which we deny ourselves. Faith says, "Lord, you don't owe me anything; I, on the other hand, owe you everything." When we exercise our faith in God we submissively and sincerely acquiesce to God and his will, whatever that will may be. Faith does not dictate what God's will is. The spiritual posture of the child of God is one of quiet expectancy, ready to receive from God whatever he in his infinite wisdom and mercy deigns to give, or for that matter, to withhold.

In the absence of an explicit biblical promise, it is little short of arrogance to pray to God as if we already know what he wills. If the *Bible* does not say God's will is that I be healed, it is insolent for *me* to say it. Merely because *we* believe or have convinced ourselves that God wants to heal us does not mean that he does. He surely *may*, but not because we have coaxed him into it by our faith. God is sovereign and free to do as he pleases and is not dependent on the moods, far less the demands, of creatures like you and me. We must never wield our faith as if it were a whip by which we compel God to respond. We do not force his will into submission to ours simply by banishing doubt from our hearts.

Dave Hunt has suggested that this notion of faith has more in common with sorcery than it does with the Bible. He describes it as follows:

> Many sincere Christians have been influenced by the sorcerer's gospel to imagine that faith has some power in itself. Once again, to them faith is not placed *in* God but is a power directed *at* God, which forces Him to do for us what we have *believed* He will do. At the very least this makes God subject to alleged "laws" that we can activate by "faith"; at worst it eliminates God from the process altogether, putting everything in our own hands and thus turning us into gods who can make anything happen by our "power of belief." If everything works according to such "law," then God is no longer sovereign and there is no place for grace. All one needs to do is to exercise this "power of belief." That is the basic idea behind sorcery.[11]

When we pray to God for healing, it is by faith in the power of *God*, not by faith in the power of faith. What we believe is not that God will do what suits our understanding of his will, but that he will do what is compatible with his character as revealed in Scripture. He is loving and therefore always has our ultimate spiritual best in mind, which may or may not involve our physical healing. He is wise and therefore not only is able to provide us with what we need even when we don't think we need it, but also knows when to withhold from us what we think we need but really don't.

To preface or conclude our prayers with the proviso "if it be Thy will" is anything but a "faith-killing statement." It is the very essence of faith, a humble confession of our creatureliness and our ignorance of the future. It is our way of acknowledging to God that we deserve nothing and that we therefore depend wholly on his goodness and greatness.

Joni Eareckson Tada

Aside from the theological problems I have mentioned, there is an immediate practical issue that must be addressed. Perhaps the best illustration of what I have in mind is the well-known case of Joni Eareckson Tada. In her book *A Step Further* she tells of a prayer meeting held some five years after the accident that left her paralyzed. Friends, family members, and church leaders gathered to pray fervently for healing. She was anointed with oil. They praised God. They believed God. Healing was claimed. They left aglow and uplifted. But Joni was still in her wheelchair. She began to ask herself:

> *Is there some sin in my life?* Well, of course, there is still sin in every Christian's life. No one is without it. But there was no area of conscious rebellion against God on my part. I was living in close fellowship with Him, keeping short accounts, confessing my sins and failures to Him daily and receiving assurances of forgiveness.[12]

After being reassured that all the biblical bases had been covered, that the procedure they followed was in conformity with biblical principles, she couldn't help but wonder, "Did I have enough faith?" Joni says it better than I ever could:

> What a flood of guilt that question brings. It constantly leaves the door open for the despairing thought: *God didn't heal me because there is something wrong with me. I must not have believed hard enough.* You can easily see how this can produce a vicious cycle: A Christian who is afflicted with some sort of physical problem asks a friend, "Do you think God would heal me if I asked Him?" "Of course He will," the friend assures him. "But you mustn't doubt. The slightest trace of doubt may prevent your being healed." So knowing that "faith comes by hearing, and hearing by the Word of God," the ill person spends hours in the Bible, reading about God's mighty power and wonderful promises, in order to strengthen his faith. Finally, he feels ready to pray. He prays by himself, with the elders of the church, at a healing service, or whatever, but he doesn't get healed. "What happened? What went wrong?" he asks. Often

he is told, "The problem isn't with God. He's always ready and waiting. The blame must be yours. You probably didn't really let your faith go and trust God all the way." Yet the poor guy *knows* he believed God in that prayer for healing more than he's ever believed God in his life.[13]

According to Joni, this is when a vicious cycle of guilt begins to swirl. When the person doesn't receive healing, doubt fills his mind: "Did God *really* want to heal me? If so, why didn't he?" Merely asking these questions leads to a weakening of his faith. He has been told that if he were strong in faith, the kind of faith that guarantees healing, he would never have wondered about God's intent in the first place. But "each unanswered prayer makes him doubt more and more, which in turn makes his chances for healing less and less! It becomes a losing battle."[14]

David Watson

Another illuminating example is the case of David Watson, a British pastor and author who died of cancer on February 18, 1984. He tells his story in *Fear No Evil*, a book he was encouraged to write chronicling his final year on this earth and his struggle with terminal illness. I knew of David Watson before word reached me of his condition. From two of his books that I had read I was aware that he was something of a driving force in the charismatic renewal in England. Even though I did not agree with all of his views, I was deeply impressed with his love for the Lord Jesus Christ. If ever there was a man of faith it was David Watson.

It is impossible to calculate how many people prayed for him all around the world. They believed that God *could* heal him, and perhaps most believed that God *would* heal him. Watson himself tells of his own struggle with faith, how he confessed and repented of all known and hidden sins. He went so far as to write letters asking forgiveness from those he had harmed or offended, as well as letters to those who had hurt and embittered him. He settled all accounts, human and divine, physical and spiritual. He prayed, he surrendered, he was anointed, and he died.

Would that we all had one-tenth the faith of David Watson. Would that we all might pray as fervently and sincerely as did those godly believers who interceded for him during that final year. Yet, notwithstanding the belief, knowledge, wants, wishes, and prayers of so great a multitude, it simply was *not* God's will that David Watson be healed. At least, not in one sense of the term. James I. Packer, in his foreword to *Fear No Evil*, puts it this way:

> David's theology led him to believe, right to the end, that God wanted to heal his body. Mine leads me rather to say that God evidently wanted David home, and healed his whole person by taking him to glory in the way that he will one day heal us all. Health and life, I would say, in the full and final sense of those words, are not what we die *out of*, but what we die *into*.[15]

Do you lose faith when you see Joni Eareckson Tada in a wheelchair or when you visit the gravesite of someone like David Watson? God certainly doesn't intend for you to. If anything our faith ought to deepen and intensify. When I see Joni serve the Lord Jesus Christ with such devotion in spite of her affliction, the true meaning of Christian "faith" begins to sink in. Her life tells me of a God who leads us in spiritual triumph, not necessarily *out of* physical disability, but *through* it. And when I know that David Watson lives now as he never lived before, my confidence in the God of my salvation grows as I myself look with anxious expectation for the day of ultimate healing.

5

IS THERE A DOCTOR
IN THE HOUSE?

During the twelve years that my wife and I lived in Dallas, Texas, we made numerous trips north on U.S. 75, through the eastern hills of Oklahoma to Tulsa, where her parents reside. It is a drive of about five hours and often proved wearisome to our young daughter. Toward the end of the trip she would begin to ask, at five-minute intervals, "Daddy, when are we going to be there?" "Not much longer, honey," I would respond. "Do you see the tall buildings up ahead?" She would smile and sit back in her seat; at least for another five minutes!

The "tall buildings up ahead" were not the skyscrapers of downtown Tulsa, but the Oral Roberts City of Faith Medical and Research Center. Featuring a 62-story clinic flanked on either side by a 30-story hospital and a 20-story research building, this remarkable complex on the south side of Tulsa has captured the attention of many a weary traveller.

Faith and Medicine

The City of Faith symbolizes far more than the end of a long drive to Tulsa. It represents what Rodney Clapp calls "an all-out fusion of science and religion."[1] The 777-bed hospital and research center were constructed specifically to provide for the joint ministry of healing through faith and modern science. Although his early days as a tent-revivalist may not reflect it, Oral Roberts is now the leading advocate among charismatics of the compatibility of divine healing and modern medicine. The patients in his hospital are attended to daily by both a physician and a prayer partner. Roberts himself made no apologies when he recently underwent surgery to repair a torn rotator cuff in his shoulder.

Roberts is not alone in his desire to see faith and physicians working in tandem. I recently read the story of Dr. Jim Hayes, a family physician who practices in St. Augustine, Florida. Dr. Hayes not only prescribes medication and performs surgery but also lays hands on the sick, prays for their healing, and commands evil spirits to leave their bodies. He even describes his own healing. "My condition," he explains, "was medically termed chronic lumbosacral strain with a locked facet syndrome, which means the vertebrae in the lower back region had become fused because of scar tissue."[2] Dr. Hayes goes on to tell how he was totally healed of this condition at a "Healing Explosion" in Jacksonville, Florida.[3]

The relationship between the charismatic movement and medical science, however, has not always been a polite one. If there is an emerging alliance between the two, and that remains to be seen, it is an uneasy and tenuous one. Ever since healing became a prominent feature among charismatic ministers, physicians have been looked upon with more than a healthy dose of suspicion.

Faith Versus Medicine

Consider the example of John Alexander Dowie, who has been called "the father of healing revivalism in America."[4] Coming from Australia, he settled in Chicago in 1893. He purchased some land 30 miles north of the city hoping to establish his own "Zion." Dowie made no bones about his disdain for medical science, at least as far as Christians were concerned. He is an excellent example of the extreme element in the early days of Pentecostalism in America. His emphasis on divine healing through faith was so intense, says Bruce Barron, that "he loudly lumped doctors, drugs and devils in the same category and outlawed all three of them in his city."[5]

Another case in point is Jack Coe, who was also a highly influential figure in the early days of the healing revival. Coe, like Dowie, staunchly opposed the use of medicine and physicians. If God was willing to heal, as Coe insisted he was, reliance on any other remedy was tantamount to disbelief. Consequently, Coe's premature death from polio in 1957 constituted what David Harrell has described as "perhaps the greatest shock in the history of the healing revival."[6]

Undoubtedly one of the most vocal opponents of modern medical science was the late Hobart Freeman, pastor of Faith Assembly in Indiana. His story is also the most tragic.[7] Freeman's antagonism toward medicine was unbridled. In one place he wrote:

> To claim healing for the body and then to continue to take medicine is not following our faith with corresponding actions. One should settle the matter beforehand; if we have faith that God will keep His Word and heal us, then we will not need to keep our medicines and remedies around "just in case."[8]

Freeman went so far as to forbid his followers to wear eyeglasses. Some members of Faith Assembly who discarded their glasses, having "claimed" their healing, reportedly were still able to pass their driving tests. But as Bruce Barron says, "They have still been seen squinting as they read their Bibles."[9] Ironically, while Freeman preached his extreme view, he himself was anything but the model of good health.

> In his case the disease was visible to all who saw him: polio, suffered when he was a child, forced him to wear a special riser for his withered right leg. According to Faith Assembly's explanation, the healing of this leg "has been claimed by faith, but the manifestation has not occurred yet." An alternate explanation also given was that the limp was an example of " 'Job's trials' designed to enrich [Freeman's] ministry." No one within Faith Assembly ever dared to suggest that Freeman might be guilty of the same lack of faith to which he attributed the illnesses and deaths of his parishioners.[10]

Of course, the ultimate tragedy in this story is that by the end of 1984 the number of documented deaths at Faith Assembly had risen to 90. Virtually all of these victims could have survived had they received medical help. The majority of those who died were infants and young children. On December 8, 1984, Freeman died at the age of 64 from bronchopneumonia and heart failure, having refused to seek medical treatment for himself.

One might hope that such an attitude toward medical science is rare and isolated. Unfortunately, it is not. The September 9, 1984 edition of *The Dallas Morning News* carried the story of Thomas and Connie Sorrell, whose four-year-old daughter, Vickie, died of Rocky Mountain spotted fever. The Sorrells, lifelong members of the Church of God, were charged with second degree manslaughter for not providing her with medical treatment. The Rev. Leslie Busbee, pastor of the Guthrie, Oklahoma, church was quoted as saying:

> We do not have a church law against doctors. But we have strong sentiments against medicine. When you look at medical science full in the face, there is no guarantee. But when you trust in the Lord through prayer, you are in contact with someone who can never make a mistake. We have one case where a child dies, but we have hundreds of cases where children have been healed.[11]

Sadly, I have in my files numerous other articles documenting cases similar to that of the Sorrells'.

Faith Tolerant of Medicine

The majority of charismatics seem to have taken a more modified stance on the use of physicians and medicine. They generally acknowledge that on occasion God may well inspire someone to stop taking medication or to disregard their symptoms. But this is not to suggest that God always works that way.[12] According to Barron, whereas they support the use of doctors, "sometimes in the same breath they seem to suggest that doctors should serve only as a stopgap measure for Christians until they reach a higher level of faith."[13] Unfortunately, this places the believer in the unenviable position of appearing spiritually weak and immature should he seek medical assistance. Going to a doctor is not openly condemned, but it does seem to be an unspoken measure of one's faith in God or lack thereof. In such a case "subtle peer pressure could compel the sick to claim their healing and receive admiration for their faith rather than go to the doctor and risk implicit disapproval."[14]

The fact remains that no matter how loudly charismatics declare their appreciation for the medical profession, they retain a basic disaffection for it. One senses this in a statement such as that made by Hugh Jeter. "Although the Lord did not condemn physicians, He did not send anyone to them for help. He did not need to. He had, and still has, 'all power in heaven and in earth.'"[15] Faint praise indeed!

What to Make of a Bad Prognosis

One aspect of a physician's task that comes in for special criticism is that of prognosis. John Wimber, for example, who is fast becoming the most popular charismatic author and speaker both in America and in England, says that doctors can hinder healing by describing the situation "in a way that convinces the patient that he will not get better."[16] Wimber suggests that an obstacle to healing is created when physicians inform their patients of their odds for recovery. Consequently, "in many instances the Holy Spirit heals the physical damage only after the power of the doctor's words is broken."[17] Blaine Cook also believes that there is a negative force in a physician's words. If a doctor says "you have terminal cancer; nothing more can be done," it may give rise to a "defeated attitude."[18] That no doubt is possible, and I certainly would not endorse a calloused and insensitive bedside manner. But I'm convinced that this is rare in the medical community. The vast majority of physicians are caring and sensitive people who take into consideration both the feelings of the patient and his need (and right) to know the gravity of his condition.

A good example of some bad thinking on this issue is found in the following statements by Colin Urquhart.

> Imagine that two Christians, both born-again men, receive an identical prognosis from the doctor: they have cancer and are expected to live for only three months. The first receives the news passively. "Thank you, doctor. Can nothing be done?" When he is told that medical treatment would be of no avail, he leaves the surgery believing he is under sentence of death. He has received the cancer in his spirit as well as having it in

his body. Subsequently, he may pray because he realises God is able to heal. But he has a real faith battle on his hands because of the double healing he needs. He believes not only the cancer, but the doctor's prognosis.[19]

The second man, says Urquhart, hears an identical verdict, but his response is quite different. This man replies:

"No, I will not die within three months because by the stripes of Jesus I have been healed." He meets the situation with active, positive and definite faith. He refuses to accept or believe the fact of the cancer in his spirit, although he knows the fact of it in his body.[20]

I'm not sure why Urquhart thinks these men should have listened to a physician in the first place. If the first man was wrong in believing the medical accuracy of the prognosis, why did he seek the doctor's counsel at all? Urquhart suggests that the man is weak in faith and has little hope for healing because he "believes . . . the doctor's prognosis." But why shouldn't he believe it? Does he have reason to think the doctor was lying? And why should Urquhart conclude that this man's confidence in the skill of his physician means "he has received the cancer in his spirit as well as having it in his body"?

While I admire the second man's will to live, I see no biblical basis for his assurance that he shall. What happens if he *does* die? Were the "stripes of Jesus" inadequate to secure his healing? If not, then the failure must be in the faith of the man himself. But if *his* faith is at fault, how does he differ at all from the first man? And what does it mean to say "he refuses to accept or believe the fact of the cancer in his spirit, although he knows the fact of it in his body"? If the cancer is truly in his body, why is it contrary to Christian faith to acknowledge that reality?

A Christian Response

What ought to be the proper response of a Christian in a situation like this? I believe he first ought to thank his physician for speaking honestly and realistically. If he was determined not to believe what his doctor was going to say because of his faith in what he believed Jesus would do, he should never have wasted his time and money in seeking medical assistance. If it is a lack of faith in God to believe the physician's prognosis, it was a lack of faith in God to consult him in the first place. But having done so he should be grateful for knowing his actual physical condition, and should readily concede that as far as medical science is concerned, his earthly life may well be at its end. He should then pray: "Dear Heavenly Father, I know that you can do what medical science cannot. I humbly request that you destroy this cancer and restore me to full health, that I might live fully to your glory on this earth. But if you should choose not to do so, my faith and confidence in your goodness and greatness remains constant. If it is indeed your will, then I rejoice in the prospect of my ultimate healing and the expectation of seeing my Savior face to face. Thy will be done."

Perhaps the problem here is the failure to realize that not all healing is miraculous, in the technical sense of that term. In fact, most healing is not. Dr. Paul Brand reminds us that God has endowed the human body with the remarkable power of healing itself. For example:

> An infected wound is red and swollen with pus: the redness comes from an emergency blood supply rushing white cells and agents of repair to the scene and the pus, composed of lymph fluids and dead cells, gives stark and dramatic evidence of cellular warfare being fought. Similarly, a fever represents the body's effort to circulate blood more quickly and also create a hostile environment for some bacteria. Vomiting coordinates scores of muscles in a dramatic reversal of their normal processes: designed to push food down through the intestine, they now regroup in order to violently expel the food along with toxins and unwelcome invaders that have accumulated in the stomach. All these irritations, which most of us view with alarm and even disgust, reveal the orderly progress of the healing body.[21]

When a broken bone is set, the body itself ultimately provides the calcium necessary for permanent healing. A surgeon's incision is safe only because the body repairs itself by supplying new cells and tissue. Whereas we tend to focus on those instances when the body succumbs to disease or injury, Brand points out that "for each breakdown there are hundreds of examples of microbes slaughtered before they could cause damage, of tuberculosis patches isolated in the lungs, and of breast cancers strangled by the body's own defenses."[22]

In every case the body's recuperative power is traceable to its Creator. If an aspirin relieves a headache, it is not to the pharmaceutical company that ultimate gratitude is due. God supplied nature with the ingredients in aspirin, and it is God who created, sustains, and enables the body to respond positively to its medicinal properties. He is the one to thank for the successful surgical transplant of a kidney or for relief from depression or a head cold. It is God who deserves praise for the polio vaccine that enables children to walk, and for the corrective powers of eyeglasses that enable us to see, and for penicillin and other so-called "miracle drugs" that enable us to live to his glory. All genuine healing, whether miraculous or not, is ultimately the work of God.

Therefore, the question is not so much whether God heals, but how. If we believe God is Lord over all creation and that every natural, physical, and chemical process is subject to his will, surely whatever healing comes via those means is no less "divine" than those healings we refer to as "miraculous." God is no less deserving of glory and honor when he destroys cancer cells through radiation treatment than when he does it directly, apart from some secondary instrumentality.

So the next time you are sick, pray that God will use all the means at his disposal to heal you. Then thank him for your physician, as you dial the phone to set up an appointment.

ADDENDUM
PSYCHOSOMATIC ILLNESS

The capacity of the human body to heal itself, as we have seen, is a marvelous gift of God. But what about the *mind?* We often hear people refer to the power of "mind over body." Is there any truth to it? Does the mind exercise an influence over the body? If so, what relevance does this have for the subject of healing? Dr. Paul Brand has some important and insightful comments in this regard that I believe are worthy of your attention. The following material has been taken from the article by Dr. Brand and Philip Yancey, "A Surgeon's View of Divine Healing," *Christianity Today*, November 25, 1983, 18-19, and is used by permission.

> Skeptical scientists and physicians use the word "psycho-somatic" to explain away reports of supernatural healings, implying the particular ailment healed was due more to auto-suggestion than to any physical "miracle." They point out that healings occur in certain groupings of diseases: neurasthenia, bursitis, arthritis, lameness, deafness, allergies, migraine headaches.
>
> Although divine healing seems to work best among selective afflictions, it does attract enthusiastic testimonials. Thousands of people take the trouble to write national television programs claiming deliverance from suffering; we cannot simply dismiss their reports.
>
> It does not diminish my respect for God's power in the slightest to realize that he primarily works through faculties of the mind to summon up new resources of healing in a person's body. The word "psychosomatic" carries no derogatory connotations for me. It derives from two Greek words, *psyche* and *soma*, which mean simply "mind" or "soul," and "body." Such diseases and their apparent cures demonstrate the incredible power of the mind in affecting the rest of the body.
>
> Let me illustrate the mind's power with a few examples recently documented by modern science:
>
> • The mind can effectively control pain. This can be accomplished by simple mental discipline or by "flooding the gates" of the nervous system with distracting noises or additional sensations (e.g., acupuncture). I saw impressive evidence of pain control while in India, where Hindu fakirs would unflinchingly walk on coals, sleep on nails, and string themselves up on poles with ropes pulling on meat hooks through their backs.
>
> • In the placebo effect, faith in simple sugar pills stimulates the mind to control pain and even heal some disorders. In

some experiments among those with terminal cancer, morphine was an effective painkiller in two-thirds of patients, but placebos were equally effective in half of those! The placebo tricks the mind into believing relief has come, and the body responds accordingly. Placebos also show curative powers in areas other than in pain control; they can actually stimulate the fight against disease.

• Through biofeedback, people can train themselves to direct bodily processes that previously were thought involuntary. They can control blood pressure, heart rate, brain waves, and even vary the temperature in their hands by as much as 14 degrees.

• In primitive cultures, shamans use a technique called "boning." The shaman points a "magical" bone at a person accused of some crime, and the person will contort and writhe in pain, and die in a few hours. The only physical "cause" of death is the power of suggestion.

• Under hypnosis, 20 percent of patients can be induced to lose consciousness of pain so completely that they can undergo surgery without anesthetics. Some patients have even cured their own warts under hypnosis. The hypnotist suggests the idea, and the body performs a remarkable feat of skin renovation and construction, involving the cooperation of thousands of cells in a mental-directed process not otherwise attainable.

• In a false pregnancy, a woman believes so strongly in her pregnant condition that her mind directs an extraordinary sequence of activities: it increases hormone flow, enlarges breasts, suspends menstruation, induces morning sickness, and even prompts labor contractions. All this occurs even though there is no "physical cause"—that is, no fertilization and growing fetus inside.

Brain researchers have recently received Nobel Prizes for discovering the mechanisms behind some of these mind-body connections. The brain produces an array of chemical neurotransmitters called endorphins that can control pain and affect body systems, some of which are hundreds of times more potent than morphine.

Simultaneously, many researchers have explored how external factors, such as stress, can have profound effects on body systems. People who are unemployed or recently widowed have much higher susceptibility to disease. People who take quiet times during the day and force themselves to relax seem to develop a control of stress that brings them to greater health. All of these findings, which are far too numerous and complex to explore in this article, point to the fact that the mind can be a powerful channel for directing physical healing, or its failure.

Is this mental-directed healing the mechanism that results in so many claims of healing from faith healing ministries? It seems very probable. The suffering person may well focus hope and faith and trust to such a degree that the physical body responds with true recovery. The mind is a powerful force, and God can use it for his good purposes.

Notice that Dr. Brand believes "many" claims of healing are traceable to the influence of mind over body. I am inclined to agree with him, though this is not to suggest that "all" healings are of this order. At least *I* make no such suggestion.

Nevertheless, I concur with Dr. Brand that the power of belief and expectation is immense. When we reflect on this in the light of chapter 5, there is even greater cogency in Dr. Brand's observations. You will recall that most faith healers insist that if healing is going to occur, a person must first bring himself to believe that God not only wants to heal him but *will* heal him. Often they go so far as to say that he must believe that God *already has* healed him. When this is combined with the high-level emotional atmosphere generated in many healing services, as well as the dynamic and persuasive personality of the healer himself (or herself), the "mental stage" is set for what may prove to be remarkable results.

In saying this, however, I do not want to be misunderstood. I do not mean to imply that God cannot or will not intervene directly and supernaturally to effect a cure, even of so-called "organic" diseases. Both Dr. Brand and Dr. William A. Nolen, author of *Healing: A Doctor in Search of a Miracle* (New York: Random House, 1974), are somewhat skeptical about the miraculous healing of organic afflictions (the latter more so than the former). I am not. But I do believe that if God does move in this manner, he does so rarely, and that the vast number of reported healings in our day may be explained on other grounds.

6

SATAN, SIN, AND SUFFERING

There is no getting around the fact that Job is an embarrassment, an enigma, an inexplicable glitch in the "God-wants-you-healthy-and-wealthy" philosophy of many contemporary charismatics. Oral Roberts has become famous for telling his audience with all the assurance he can muster, "Something *good* is going to happen to you today!" Job may beg to differ.

The story of this Old Testament figure is truly remarkable, and yet many have failed to grasp the significance of his suffering. That may be due in part to the deeply theological character of the book of Job itself. The issues in it are not easily digested. But I am persuaded that the principal cause for confusion is its portrait of God. If God is good and great, as we believe he is, how can he stand idly by and permit a righteous man like Job to suffer so horribly?[1] Unable to answer this question, people rashly jump to the conclusion that either Job was *not* righteous or Satan was ultimately responsible for what happened.

The great majority of faith healers today consistently attribute sickness and suffering to either the devil or human disobedience. Satan and sin alone account for ill health and financial destitution. God is the opponent, never the origin, of adversity such as Job experienced. "Know this once for all," declares Norvel Hayes: "all bad things that come to visit you are from the devil—*all* bad things! They come from hell—not from heaven."[2] You can readily see that Job just doesn't fit this mold. In fact, he shatters it. Let's consider more closely this man and his suffering.

Job and His Trial
The first and most important thing we learn about Job is that he was a blameless and upright man, who feared God and turned

47

away from evil (Job 1:1, 8). It is as if the author wants us to understand right from the beginning that Job's suffering is not the consequence of his sin. That is not to say Job was perfect, for all through
the book he acknowledges that all men are born sinners. But by
God's gracious enablement Job pursued a life of purity. In fact, his
concern for righteousness extended beyond his own life to that of
his children. We are told in 1:5 that he would rise up early in the
morning and offer burnt sacrifices for them, saying, "Perhaps my
sons have sinned and cursed God in their hearts."

Satan was at a loss. Job was a complete puzzle to him. He didn't
doubt that Job was obedient and upright—there was no mistaking
his godliness. But the devil just couldn't bring himself to believe
that anyone would want to be holy *for nothing*. The only thing left
for him to do was to launch an assault against Job's motives.
Though he could hardly question Job's righteousness, he did
wonder about the reason for it. His diabolical conclusion was that
Job served God for what he could get out of him. Job's piety, rea-
soned the devil, must be a calculated effort to milk God of his gifts.
"Take away the pay and he'll quit the job," he thought. You see,
Satan was persuaded that worship is fundamentally selfish—nothing more than a man-made device to flatter God into generosity.
Therefore, if God's generosity were cut off, Job's praise would turn
to cursing. Consequently, when Satan came before God, he said:

> Does Job fear God for nothing? Hast Thou not made a hedge
> about him and his house and all that he has, on every side? Thou
> hast blessed the work of his hands, and his possessions have
> increased in the land. But put forth Thy hand now and touch
> all that he has; he will surely curse Thee to Thy face (1:9-11).

In order to prove to Satan that Job's devotion was not tied to
God's gifts, the Lord sovereignly permitted Satan to afflict him.
The Sabeans (1:15) and Chaldeans (1:17) attacked, killing his
livestock and animals. Even his sons and daughters were slain
(1:18-19). Job's immediate reaction makes sense to most of us. He
arose, tore his clothes in anguish, shaved his head, and fell to the
ground (1:20)! But just when you expect to hear him whine and
complain and ask "Why me, Lord?" he began to *worship*! That's

right, *he worshipped!* His love, faith, and commitment to God did not end when his suffering began. He proved immediately to the devil and to us that his devotion was not dependent on a continuous flow of gifts and good times. God is worthy of his devotion because he is *God*, period. Job's words of praise are as astounding as they are brief: "And he said, 'Naked I came from my mother's womb, and naked I shall return there. The Lord gave and the Lord has taken away. Blessed be the name of the Lord'" (1:21).

Note well that Job does not say, "The Lord gave and the *Sabeans* have taken away!" or "The Lord gave and the *Chaldeans* have taken away!" Nor even does he say, "The Lord gave and *Satan* has taken away!" Rather, he acknowledged God as the cause of *all* outcomes, both plenty and poverty. As Francis Anderson expressed it: "Job sees only the hand of God in these events. It never occurs to him to curse the desert brigands, to curse the frontier guards, to curse his own stupid servants, now lying dead for their watchlessness. All secondary causes vanish. It was the Lord who gave; it was the Lord who removed; and in the Lord alone must the explanation of these strange happenings be sought."[3]

The exegetical extremes to which some people will go in order to evade the clear teaching of this book are incredible. Consider, for example, the interpretation of Frederick K. Price, one of this country's leading faith healers and charismatic authors. He first insists that Job suffered because he sinned. It was *Job*, says Price, not God, who lowered the hedge around himself (cf. 1:10). "As long as Job walked in *faith*, the wall—the hedge—was *up*. But when he started walking in *unbelief* and *doubt* the hedge was pulled down. JOB PULLED IT DOWN."[4] Price draws this remarkable conclusion in the complete absence of any text asserting or implying that Job lived in sinful unbelief and doubt. Furthermore, the protective hedge was put around Job by *God* and therefore could only be removed by God, as 1:12 clearly implies. Moreover, if Job was living in sinful unbelief and doubt, as Price suggests, Satan would have lost his reason for afflicting him. Satan's desire was to prove that Job's *obedience* was conditioned upon the blessings God had bestowed. He wanted to prove that God, in and of himself, was not worthy of Job's praise. If Job was living in disobedience, doubt, and unbelief, what reason would Satan have had for carrying through with his scheme? Also, Price's interpretation is flatly contradicted by what God himself said of Job in 2:3. After Job had suffered the loss of all his material wealth, God said to Satan: "Have you considered My servant Job? For there is no one like him on the earth, a blameless and upright man fearing God and turning away from evil. And he *still* holds fast his integrity, although you incited Me against him, to ruin him without cause." Clearly, Price's attempt to impugn Job's character is a desperate grasping at straws.

As if that were not enough, Price goes on to argue that Job was confused and mistaken when he uttered the words of 1:21. "The Lord gave and the Lord has taken away," says Price, "is not a true statement. God didn't do that to Job. Satan did it. But Job thought that God did it. . . . Job didn't rashly accuse God, but he didn't know anybody else to *put it on*, so he said the Lord did it."[5] But again, there is no indication in this passage that Job was mistaken. Indeed, 1:12 clearly implies that it was in fact God who ultimately controlled Satan's access to Job. And what will Price do with 2:3, in which God tells the devil that Job "still holds fast his integrity, although you incited Me [God] against him, to ruin him without cause"? Surely Price would not want to argue that God was confused about the source of Job's suffering! And what of Job's wife? Although her counsel to "curse God and die" (2:9) was rash and ill-conceived, it at least reveals her conviction that God was the ultimate source of Job's calamities.

Job was obviously persuaded of the same thing. What he said in 1:21 following the first series of tragedies is repeated in 2:10 following the second. Job's response to his wife is clear and unequivocal: "You speak as one of the foolish women speaks. Shall we indeed accept good from God and not accept adversity?" Only theological prejudice can sidestep the exegetical facts. God had given Job all he owned and God, through the instrumentality of Satan, had taken it away. But the testing of this remarkable man didn't stop with his wealth. It reached also to his health.

When we turn to chapter 2, we discover that Satan, in accordance with his character, was not satisfied with Job's financial and material deprivation. Nothing short of an all-out assault on his body, his flesh and bones, would quench his sadistic thirst. "So the Lord said to Satan, 'Behold, he [Job] is in your power, only spare his life'" (2:6). What happened to Job next is almost too gruesome to describe.

Satan didn't waste a moment's time. He "went out from the presence of the Lord, and smote Job with sore boils from the sole of his foot to the crown of his head" (2:7). Someone has suggested that Job suffered from leprosy, but we can't be sure. However, knowing Satan as we do, we can be certain that these "sore boils" were indescribably painful and grievous. Satan has never been one to show mercy on anyone, least of all one of God's children.

The disease is said to have covered his entire body (2:7) and led to intolerable itching (2:8; the potsherd was probably used to scrape off pus from the sores). His appearance was disfigured, leaving him unrecognizable to his friends (2:12; cf. 19:19). He suffered a loss of appetite (3:24a), depression (3:24b-26; 7:16), and sleeplessness (7:4). When he did sleep, he experienced nightmares (7:14). He was afflicted with festering sores and broken skin (7:5), scabs that blackened and peeled (30:30), high fever (30:30), excessive weeping and burning in the eyes (16:16), putrid breath (19:17), an emaciated body (17:7; 19:20), and chronic pain (30:17). In his agony he took his place on the dung heap ("the ashes," 2:9), where dogs scavenged for food among the corpses and refuse.

Lessons From Job's Ordeal

What does God intend for us to learn from Job's experience? Surely he is telling us, among other things, that obedience does not guarantee we will experience good health and great wealth. We may, and if we do we should humbly thank God for his gifts. But then again we may not, and if we do not we should humbly thank God for what little we do have. After all, we don't deserve to have anything in the first place. The mere fact that Job was alive at all was an act of sovereign grace.

We also learn that not all special sickness is the result of some special sin. Job was afflicted in spite of his righteousness. He feared and obeyed God before, during, and after his suffering, to the obvious dismay of the devil back then and to the discomfort of health-and-wealth advocates in our own day.

Yet another lesson we learn from Job's experience is the peril of trying to read providence. It seems as if all of us are by nature inclined to draw moral conclusions from physical events. But apart from what the Bible says, we simply don't know the reasons for tragedies and triumphs. In the absence of an inspired biblical interpretation of an event, an event is just an event. We don't know if it is a sign of God's delight or his displeasure, or for that matter, either one. Solomon once said:

> Man does not know whether it will be love or hatred; anything awaits him. It is the same for all. There is one fate for the righteous and for the wicked; for the good, for the clean, and for the unclean; for the man who offers a sacrifice and for the one who does not sacrifice. As the good man is, so is the sinner; as the swearer is, so is the one who is afraid to swear. This is an evil in all that is done under the sun, that there is one fate for all men (Eccles. 9:1b-3a).

Of course he was not saying that morality is unimportant; far less that the believer is unsure whether God loves him or not. We are always assured of God's tender compassion for his children. What Solomon meant is that often you can't tell that God loves his own merely by observing what befalls them in life. The righteous suffer and die just as the wicked do. Prosperity is no more a sure sign of God's favor than adversity is of his fury. Solomon's advice is this: "In the day of prosperity be happy, but in the day of adversity consider—God has made the one as well as the other so that man may not discover anything that will be after him" (Eccles. 7:14).

If you do not agree with Solomon, I encourage you to put him to the test. Go to the nearest hospital and ask to see a list of the patients. Most hospital admittance forms have a box or a blank space to be filled in that is marked, "religious preference" or "church denomination." What you will find in *every* hospital are roughly equal numbers of Christians and non-Christians, believers and atheists, Methodists and Baptists, Catholics and charismatics. The children of God are not exclusively favored by providence; nor are the children of the devil exclusively harmed by it. Christians get cancer and die just like non-Christians. Pagans are often more wealthy than the faithful. We all must come to grips with the fact that in this sinful, fallen world justice does not always prevail, the good are not always rewarded, and the wicked often prosper. As Solomon has said:

> The race is not to the swift, and the battle is not to the warriors, and neither is bread to the wise, nor wealth to the discerning, nor favor to men of ability; for time and chance overtake them all. Moreover, man does not know his time; like fish caught in a treacherous net, and birds trapped in a snare, so the sons of men are ensnared at an evil time when it suddenly falls on them (Eccles. 9:11-12).

When Job's friends approached him as he sat naked upon the dung heap, deprived of all material wealth, disfigured by the festering sores that covered his body, their reaction is probably like ours: "Boy, you must have *really* messed things up this time!" No, Job hadn't "messed things up," and neither had God. Nor had Satan been permitted to do anything beyond what God had ordained. So be very careful, dear friend, before you interpret providence either for yourself or someone else. When Scripture is silent, we should be silent also.

There are numerous other insights to be gained from Job's experience, but one in particular stands out above all the rest. The clearest explanation of it is provided by Joni Eareckson Tada as she struggled to come to terms with her own suffering. It is lengthy, but right on target. Read it prayerfully.

> Strange as it may seem, it appears God often not only allows, but actually insures that His children undergo and endure long periods of real difficulty. Not only that, but He seems to be hurting His own cause by letting this take place within plain view of unbelievers who scoff at Christianity. Not one embarrassing detail escapes the eyes of these scorners as they jeer, "Look at how this so-called loving God treats His devoted followers!"
>
> But wait. As we continue observing, we notice something unusual. These Christians, on whom God has sent trial after trial, refuse to complain. Rather than shake rebellious fists at

heaven, and rather than curse the One who allows them such misery, they respond with praise to their Creator.

At first the world mocks. "It's only a phase," they assure themselves. "Just wait." But as the trials continue and the Christians refuse to "curse God and die," the watching world is forced to swallow its own words and eventually drop its jaw in amazed disbelief.

Thus, *God has shown one of the most effective ways in which suffering can bring glory to Himself—it demonstrates His ability to maintain the loyalty of His people even when they face difficult trials.* If being a Christian brought us nothing but ease and comfort, the world wouldn't learn anything very impressive about our God. "Big deal," men would say. "Anybody can get a following by waiting on people hand and foot." [Isn't this precisely what Satan said to God about Job?] But when a Christian shows faith and love for his Maker in spite of the fact that, on the surface, it looks as if he's been forgotten, it does say something impressive. It shows the scoffers that our God is worth serving even when the going gets tough. It lets a skeptical world know that what the Christian has is real.[6]

Was Job's God worth serving, even when the going got tough? Satan didn't think so. But Job did. So do I.

Addendum

Joni on Job and His God

The portrait of God in the book of Job is unsettling to a great many people. They feel compelled to conclude that God is either too weak to deliver Job from his suffering or too wicked to care. Of course, both conclusions are blasphemous. If God is not omnipotent as well as benevolent, he is not God. So how do we account for what we read in this book of the Bible? For reasons that are obvious, I believe there is someone far better qualified than I to answer that question. What follows is taken from Joni's book *A Step Further* (Grand Rapids: Zondervan, 1978), 176-80. I hope this excerpt will encourage you to read the entire book.

If anyone ever needed to understand the "why" behind his condition, it was Job. His family had been killed, his property ruined and stolen, and his body inflicted with boils. Not until the last five chapters of the book does God finally walk on-stage to answer the questions and challenges of Job and his friends. And when he does, do you know what reason God gives Job for all the suffering he has experienced? None. Not a word! He doesn't sit Job down and say, "Listen carefully while I give you the inside story on why I've let you go through all of this. You see, My plan is. . . ." In fact, so far is God from an-swering Job's questions that He says, "Stand up, Job. I've got a few questions to ask *you*!"

For the next four chapters God does nothing but describe in detail the awesome majesty of His own works in nature, and then asks Job if he can match them. The Lord paints vivid word pictures of the creation of the world, the vastness of the stars and space, the might of the ox, the majesty of the horse, the miracle of animal instincts and the way earth provides food for every living thing. "But of course you know all this!" God mocks Job, "For you were born before it was all created, and you are so very experienced!" (Job 38:21, LB).

I could almost feel Job cringing as God spoke to him. (I was cringing myself). *Why put Job on the spot?* I thought. All those descriptions of God's wisdom and power in nature were cer-tainly interesting. But what did they have to do with Job's trials? Job never claimed he had created the world. He never said he could explain the habits of wild animals. Why was God talking about that? Job hadn't pretended to know all the mysteries of weather cycles and birth and life. All he wanted was for God to help him understand the death of his family, the loss of his property, and the boils all over his body.

I continued reading. More nature scenes. More descriptions of God's greatness. More taunts from God like "Do you know how mountain goats give birth? . . . Can you shout to the clouds and make it rain? . . . Do you realize the extent of the earth? . . . Tell Me about it if you know!"

It still seemed so confusing. But as I came to chapter forty, some light began to dawn. God finally asked Job a question that seemed to focus in on what He had been driving at all along. "Do you still want to argue with the Almighty! Or will you yield? Do you—God's critic—have the answers? . . . Stand up like a man and brace yourself for battle. Let me ask you a question, and give me the answer. Are you going to discredit my justice and condemn me, so that you can say you are right?" (Job 40:1, 7-8, LB).

So that was it! God understood that when Job demanded "Why?" he was really asking God to be accountable to him. It seems so innocent, but in a sense, to insist on such answers from God is to set oneself over God. How absurd! We, like Job, often think God is not treating us fairly. We act as if there were some imaginary court in the sky where God must answer to something called "fairness." But what we forget is that God Himself *is* the court; and He invented fairness. What could we possibly measure His fairness against? What He does is as fair as you can get.

Look at God's awesome wisdom and power demonstrated by His marvelous works of creation. How could such a God be answerable to a puny mortal like Job, who couldn't begin to fathom God's infinite greatness? As God said in Jeremiah 49:19, "Who is like Me, and who will summon Me into court?" It was as if God were saying, "Job, if you can't even understand the way I do things in the natural world, what gives you a right to question Me in the spiritual realm, which is even harder to understand?

When Job realized this, all he could say was, "I am nothing—how could I ever find the answers? I lay my hand upon my mouth in silence. I have said too much already" (Job 40:4-5, LB).

What made Job feel this way? He got his first glimpse of who God really is. All his life he had worshipped God, but for the first time he saw God as He really is, not just his own limited concept of Him. Job put it like this: "I had heard about you before, but now I have seen you, and I loathe myself and repent in dust and ashes" (Job 42:5, LB).

My thoughts turned away from Job's situation and back to my own. I was grateful for the things I had been able to see from God's point of view. But, like Job, I still had unanswered questions. What about the things God hadn't revealed? How had I handled them?

Immediately I was convicted. The Bible tells us our God is so trustworthy that we are to throw our confidence on Him, not leaning on our own limited understanding (Prov. 3:5). God has already proved how much His love can be trusted by sending Christ to die for us. Wasn't that enough? Not for me. I always wanted to be on the inside looking out—sitting with the Lord up in the control tower instead of down on the confusing ground level. He couldn't be trusted unless I was there to oversee things!

What a low view of my Master and Creator I had held all these years! How could I have dared to assume that almighty God owed me explanations! Did I think that because I had done God the "favor" of becoming a Christian, He must now check things out with me? Was the Lord of the universe under obligation to show me how the trials of every human being fit into the tapestry of life? Had I never read Deuteronomy 29:29: "There are secrets the Lord your God has not revealed to us" (LB)?

What made me think that even if He explained all His ways to me I would be able to understand them? It would be like pouring million-gallon truths into my one-ounce brain. Why, even the great apostle Paul admitted that, though never in despair, he was often perplexed (2 Cor. 4:8). Hadn't God said, "For as the heavens are higher than the earth, so are . . . my thoughts [higher] than your thoughts" (Isa. 55:9)? Didn't one Old Testament author write, "As you do not know the path of the wind, or how the body is formed in a mother's womb, so you cannot understand the work of God, the Maker of all things" (Eccl. 11:5, NIV)? In fact, the whole book of Ecclesiastes was written to convince people like me that only God holds the keys to unlocking the mysteries of life and that he's not loaning them all out! "He has also set eternity in the hearts of men; yet they cannot fathom what God has done from the beginning to end" (Eccl. 3:11, NIV).

If God's mind was small enough for me to understand, He wouldn't be God! How wrong I had been.

I thought back to those early days of studying God's Word when the puzzle pieces of my suffering began fitting together. How sweet that first taste of wisdom was. There's nothing like seeing our difficulties from God's perspective. But what a mistake to think that I would ever be able to complete the *whole* puzzle of suffering. For wisdom is more than just seeing our problems through God's eyes—it's also trusting Him even when the pieces don't seem to fit.

7

WHY DID JESUS HEAL THE SICK?

In June of 1986 the inaugural meeting of *Charismatic Bible Ministries* was convened on the campus of Oral Roberts University in Tulsa, Oklahoma. Those who attended constituted a virtual Who's Who of the charismatic movement. What captured my immediate attention, however, wasn't so much the people at this conference as it was the huge banner draped across the back of the stage where they stood, which read, "LOVE AND UNITY THROUGH SIGNS AND WONDERS."

The phrase "signs and wonders" is especially familiar to those who follow developments in the contemporary charismatic movement. It refers to the miraculous displays of God's power that were particularly prominent in the earthly ministry of Jesus. But the participants at this gathering would insist that signs and wonders ought to be no less prominent in our ministries today. In fact, they argue that it is precisely because *Jesus* performed signs and wonders that *we* should. After all, it was he who said, whoever "believes in Me, the works that I do shall he do also; and greater works than these shall he do; because I go to the Father" (John 14:12). I'll have more to say about this passage later on, but for now I am concerned with the message on the banner.

Were love and unity the purpose for which Jesus performed signs and wonders? The biblical evidence would indicate not. Nowhere in the New Testament are we led to believe that Jesus performed miracles in order to increase love and cultivate unity among believers. Of course, Jesus encouraged love and unity, but those two virtues were not the only reason or even the necessary result of his miracles. So why *did* Jesus perform signs and wonders? What was the divine purpose in the healing of the multitudes? It seems that only by understanding God's design for the miraculous in the first century shall we be able to assess claims for the same in the twentieth. So again, let me ask the question: Why did Jesus heal the sick? As I read the New Testament, there seem to have been no fewer than five reasons for miraculous healing. Let me briefly survey them.

Authentication

Perhaps the most important reason why God healed people through Jesus was to authenticate and certify him as Messiah. Peter could hardly have been more explicit concerning this when he preached on the Day of Pentecost. He described Jesus as "a man *attested* to you by God with miracles and wonders and signs which God performed through Him in your midst" (Acts 2:22). Nicodemus revealed his understanding of this when he confessed to Jesus, "Rabbi, we know that You have come from God as a teacher; for no one can do these signs that You do unless God is with him" (John 3:2). Jesus healed the paralytic in order to prove "that the Son of Man has authority to forgive sins" (Mark 2:10). When John the Baptist was having his doubts about Jesus and wanted some evidence to confirm his identity, the Lord told his disciples, "Go and report to John the things which you hear and see: the blind receive sight and the lame walk, the lepers are cleansed and the deaf hear, and the dead are raised up, and the poor have the gospel preached to them" (Matt. 11:4-5).

On two other occasions Jesus pointed to his miraculous works as proof of his messianic identity. The works the Father has given me to accomplish, said Jesus, "the very works that I do, *bear witness* of Me, that the Father has sent Me" (John 5:26). When the Pharisees threatened to seize Jesus for claiming to be equal with God, he responded to them, "If I do not do the works of My Father, do not believe Me; but if I do them, though you do not believe Me, believe the works, that you may know and understand that the Father is in me, and I in the Father" (John 10:37-38).

God also used signs and wonders in the early church to attest or bear witness to the authenticity of the apostles. In Corinth Paul's apostolic authority had come under fire from his enemies. Therefore he wrote to the believers in the church, "The signs of a true apostle were performed among you with all perseverance, by signs and wonders and miracles" (2 Cor. 12:12). The author of the epistle to the Hebrews also referred to this purpose for the miraculous. The glorious gospel of salvation, first spoken through the Lord, "was confirmed to us by signs and wonders and by various miracles and by gifts of the Holy Spirit according to His own will" (Heb. 2:3-4).

Inauguration

Closely related to authentication is inauguration. Among the signs that the *kingdom of God* had come in the person and work of Jesus were the miracles he performed. His power to cast out demons demonstrated the presence of the kingdom (Matt. 12:28). When Jesus commissioned the Twelve to proclaim that "the kingdom of heaven is at hand" (Matt. 10:7), he empowered them to "heal the sick, raise the dead, cleanse the lepers, [and] cast out demons" (Matt. 10:8). Again, when he sent out the 70 he said, "And whatever city you enter, and they receive you, eat what is set before you; and heal those in it who are sick, and say to them, 'The kingdom of God has come near to you'" (Luke 10:8-9).

The miracles of healing and divine power were designed to signal that God was acting decisively for the salvation of his people. In Jesus the kingdom had come. Thus "the phrase 'signs and wonders' is biblical language for the revelatory events of a salvation history that had its climax in the incarnation, death, resurrection, and advent of the Spirit, leading to the birth of the Christian church."[1]

We must be especially careful at this point, lest we draw any unwarranted theological conclusions. I have in mind the tendency among many Christians to be reductionistic when it comes to evaluating claims for the miraculous. Let me explain.

When I say that the miracles of Jesus authenticate his messianic identity and signal the coming of his kingdom, I do not mean to suggest that miracles necessarily ceased forever once the new age was well under way. Contrary to the claims of some, the New Testament nowhere *reduces* the purpose of miracles solely to that of authentication and/or inauguration. Miracles certainly do function in that capacity, but no text of which I am aware *restricts* all miracles or the more spectacular spiritual gifts to that role and no other.

Some argue that since Jesus and the apostles have passed from the earthly scene, the need for miraculous gifts to attest their ministries has also passed. "But this argument stands up," says D. A. Carson, "*only* if such miraculous gifts are theologically tied *exclusively* to a role of attestation; and that is demonstrably not so. . . . The healing and other miracles of Jesus are explicitly connected not only with the *person* of Jesus, *but also with the new age he is inaugurating.*"[2] In other words, "the Spirit does not simply inaugurate the new age and then disappear; rather, he *characterizes* the new age."[3] Indeed, "the Holy Spirit, that 'other Counselor,' is in certain respects Jesus' replacement during this period between the 'already' and the 'not yet' so characteristic of New Testament eschatology; he is the means by which the Father and the Son continue to manifest themselves to believers (e.g. John 14:23)."[4]

Carson's point is well taken. On the one hand all must concede that certain spiritual gifts (such as tongues) and other miraculous displays of divine power function in ways particularly related to the onset of the present age. But on the other hand it does not follow, says Carson, that Luke (in Acts, or any other New Testament author) "expects them to cease once the period of inception has passed and the new age is under way, for the manifestations of the Spirit are tied *to the Spirit, to the new age*, fulfilling Old Testament prophecy, and not *merely* to their inception."[5]

My point is this. The question of the validity of miraculous signs and wonders in our day cannot be answered solely by an appeal to the role they played in betokening the advent of the kingdom in the first century. Whether or not certain spiritual gifts or signs and wonders are *now* operative must be determined by careful exegesis of *all* that the New Testament has to say concerning the manifold purposes for which God designed them (and D. A. Carson's book, *Showing the Spirit*, does this most effectively). Whatever decision you may come to regarding the duration of the charismata, as well as signs and wonders in general, the fact that they served to authenticate the Messiah and inaugurate his kingdom in the first century is no argument *in and of itself* against the possibility that

God may choose to employ them for other reasons in subsequent centuries, and perhaps even in our own day.

Illustration

Whenever Jesus healed the body of some physical sickness he illustrated the healing of the soul from sin. It was our Lord's way of providing us with a concrete, visible object lesson of our ultimate deliverance from the devastating effects of sin, whether in body, soul, or spirit.

This is beautifully seen in the healing of the blind man in John 9. Just as this man was physically blind from birth, so also are all men spiritually blind from birth. If this man is to receive physical sight, Jesus, who is "the light of the world" (John 9:5), must heal him. By way of analogy, if we hope to "see the kingdom of God" (John 3:3) we must be spiritually healed, that is to say, we must be born anew by the sovereign Spirit of God.

Perhaps nowhere is the illustrative design of bodily healing any more in evidence than in the case of leprosy. This dreaded disease was in a perverse sort of way perfectly suited to serve as a symbol to the Jewish mind of the radical and corrupting effects of sin in a person's life. Michael Harper explains how:

> Sin separates us from God and from one another. So does leprosy. Sin slowly rots away human life. So does leprosy. Sin is at first not easy to diagnose; it works silently and secretly. So does leprosy. Sin disfigures and distorts. So does leprosy. Sin paralyses and removes feeling and sensitivity. So does leprosy. Sin ultimately causes death. So does leprosy. It would be difficult looking at the whole range of human diseases to find a single one which more graphically describes human sinfulness than leprosy. The leper is commanded by the law to "look the part." His clothes are to be torn, his hair hung loose and he is to cry wherever he goes, "Unclean, unclean" (Lev. 13:45). Sin also leads us into loneliness and isolation. It separates us from people. The leper was commanded to live alone in a place outside the camp of Israel (Lev. 13:46).[6]

It is also interesting to observe that, with one exception (Luke 17:15), lepers are said to be "cleansed" of their disease, not "healed" (cf. Matt. 10:8). Thus, just as Jesus cleansed the body of the defilement caused by leprosy, so he will one day wholly cleanse our souls of the defilement of sin.

Glorification

The first public miracle of Jesus was the transformation of water into wine at a wedding in Cana (John 2:1-11). John tells us that "this beginning of His signs Jesus did in Cana of Galilee, and manifested His glory, and His disciples believed in Him" (John 2:11). Contrary to his disciples' suggestion that a certain man was born blind because of sin, Jesus declared, "It was neither that this man sinned, nor his parents; but it was in order that the works of God might be displayed in him" (John 9:3).

Perhaps the most explicit evidence that the miraculous was designed to glorify both the Father and the Son is the resurrection of Lazarus from the dead. As soon as Jesus received word that Lazarus was sick, he said, "This sickness is not unto death, but for the glory of God, that the Son of God may be glorified by it" (John 11:4; cf. 11:40). We see much the same thing in Matthew 15:29-31. There Jesus is described healing the multitudes of every conceivable disease. The result is "that the multitude marveled as they saw the dumb speaking, the cripple restored, and the lame walking, and the blind seeing; and they glorified the God of Israel" (Matt. 15:31).

Revelation

Miracles not only confirm that Jesus is the Christ; they also reveal what he is like. Every miracle he performed said something about his character, whether his goodness, his greatness, his love, his compassion, even his wrath (as in the cursing and withering of the fig tree). One sees this in the response of his disciples, especially on that occasion when he calmed a storm on the sea of Galilee. After Jesus had rebuked the raging waters, reducing them to a quiet submission, the disciples queried in astonishment: "What

kind of man is this, that even the winds and the sea obey Him?"
(Matt. 8:27). His deity and omnipotence were never more clearly
revealed than at that moment.

We also see in his miracles his compassion for the people. Mark
tells of one occasion when "a leper came to Him, beseeching Him
and falling on his knees before Him, and saying to Him, 'If You are
willing, You can make me clean.' And moved with compassion, He
stretched out His hand and touched him, and said to him, 'I am
willing; be cleansed'" (Mark 1:40-41). Jesus was "moved with compassion" (Matt. 20:34) for the two blind men who cried out to him
for help; and he restored their sight. Often we forget that before
Jesus fed the five thousand with only five loaves and two fish, he
"felt compassion for them, and healed their sick" (Matt. 14:14).

These, then, are the principal reasons why Jesus healed. They
are, therefore, the criteria by which all modern claims for the miraculous should be measured. Now that we have some idea *why*
Jesus healed the sick, our next task is to determine *how* and *for
whom* he did it. What were the characteristics of his healing ministry? Do the alleged healings in our day bear a resemblance to those
in his day? This is what we will be deciding in the next chapter.

8

HOW DID JESUS HEAL THE SICK?

The nature of Christ's healing work is of critical importance for our study, if only for the fact that virtually every faith healer today seeks to pattern his or her ministry after that of Jesus. It stands to reason that if Jesus is willing to heal as frequently and fully in the twentieth century as he did in the first (and most charismatics insist that he is), we should expect to see in our day the same thing we read about in the New Testament. Well, do we? The only way we can answer this question is by examining the character of Christ's healing work.

Which Diseases Did Jesus Heal?

The first thing of note in Jesus' ministry is that he healed all kinds of diseases. Matthew writes: "And Jesus was going about in all Galilee, teaching in their synagogues, and proclaiming the gospel of the kingdom, and healing every kind of disease and every kind of sickness among the people. And the news about Him went out into all Syria; and they brought to Him all who were ill, taken with various diseases and pains, demoniacs, epileptics, paralytics; and He healed them" (Matt. 4:23-24). Though Matthew was no physician, he was certain of one thing: Jesus never encountered a disease he was unable to cure. Jesus never paused to differentiate between so-called "organic" and "functional" disorders. Or, if he did recognize a difference, it obviously didn't matter. He healed them all![1]

The man Jesus healed in John 9 was not far-sighted or near-sighted or suffering from blurred vision. He was congenitally blind. Jesus healed people of chronic heart disease, deafness, leprosy, fevers, acute anterior poliomyelitis (Matt. 8:6), rheumatic disease of the spine (spondylitis ankylopoietica; Luke 13:11), fibroid tumors of the uterus (Mark 5:25-34), paralysis, epilepsy, and dropsy. And best of all, as clear proof that he could heal anyone of anything, he raised the dead to life again (Matt. 9:18-26; Luke 7:11-17; John 11:1-44). Jesus was accused of a lot of things by his enemies. But he was never once charged with filling people with false hopes concerning their physical conditions. There was never the slightest doubt in the minds of even his most bitter enemies concerning the reality and totality of the healings he performed.

How Essential Was Faith for Healing?

Another aspect of Jesus' healing ministry that calls for comment is the role of faith. It may surprise most people that rarely did Jesus heal someone in response to the faith of the afflicted individual. There were, of course, several occasions when Jesus was noticeably impressed by human faith (see Matt. 8:1-4; 9:19-22, 27-31; Mark 10:46-52). But, interestingly, at no time was anyone asked to believe that it was God's will to heal him. As far as I can tell, Jesus never suspended the healing of any person on his or her belief that Jesus was not only able but also willing to heal. When the leper bowed down before Jesus, he said, "Lord, *if* you are willing, You can make me clean" (Matt. 8:2). A number of charismatic authors would have us believe that Jesus should have rebuked the man. Recall how they define the kind of faith that is necessary for healing. Such faith believes not only that God is able but also that he is definitely *willing* to heal. To preface your request for healing, as this leper did, with the words "if you are willing" is not enough. According to some, Jesus should have instructed the leper to rephrase his words to say, "Lord, *since* you are willing, you can make me clean."

When Jesus himself asked a question of the two blind men, he said: "Do you believe I am *able* to do this?" (Matt. 9:28), not "Do you believe I am *willing* to do this?" On occasion God may well inspire a man or woman with a special faith to believe he is more than just able to heal, but also willing to do so, in that particular case. But there is no evidence that this is the norm, or that we should pray any differently than did the leper. As important as faith in Christ is, the conviction that he will heal is not always necessary in the one being healed. Often the afflicted person is not even present when the healing occurs, and some who are present are not even conscious. Frequently Jesus heals in response to the faith of a friend or relative of the ailing individual (see Matt. 8:5-13; 9:1ff.; 15:21-28; 17:14-18).

Thus the role of faith varies from one occasion to the next in the healing ministry of Jesus. The faith required by charismatics in our day bears only a faint resemblance to that described in the New Testament regarding healing.

But what about Mark 6:5-6, which says that Jesus "could do no miracle there [in Nazareth] except that He laid His hands upon a few sick people and healed them. And He wondered at their unbelief" (cf. Matt. 13:53-58)? This passage is often cited as proof that apart from faith there can be no healing. Notice, however, that the text does not inform us in what connection faith was lacking. Particularly, it does not say that Jesus could not perform miracles because they did not believe he was *willing* to do so. The context would indicate that more than likely their unbelief consisted of a refusal to acknowledge his messianic identity. The "faith" they lacked was "saving" faith. They had rejected Jesus himself, the promised messianic King. That was the nature of their unbelief. Furthermore,

> . . . it is doubtful whether Mark's "could not" is ontological or absolute, for Mark records other miracles in which the beneficiaries exhibit no faith (feeding the five thousand, stilling the storm, healing the Gadarene demoniac). The "could not" is related to Jesus' mission: just as Jesus could not turn stones to bread without violating his mission ([Matt.] 4:1-4), so he could not do miracles indiscriminately without turning his mission into a sideshow. The "lack of faith". . . of the people was doubtless a source of profound grief and frustration for Jesus . . . rather than something that stripped him of power.[2]

How Soon Did Healing Occur?

Yet another characteristic of the healings Jesus performed was their *immediacy*. Time and time again we read that, when Jesus healed, the individual was immediately and instantaneously restored to full health. When Jesus touched the leper "immediately his leprosy was cleansed" (Matt. 8:3; cf. Mark 1:42). The centurion's servant was healed of his paralysis "that very hour" (Matt. 8:13). The woman who suffered from a hemorrhage for 12 years was made well "at once" (Matt. 9:22). Other passages that explicitly mention the immediacy of healing include Matthew 15:28; 17:28; 20:34; Mark 2:12; Luke 4:39; John 4:46-54; and John 5:9.

Here we find the greatest disparity between the healing ministry of Jesus and that of modern charismatics. Keenly aware of this, charismatics have taken elaborate theological steps to explain away the problem. Francis MacNutt, for example, the author of two popular books on healing, says that the most important thing he has learned about praying for healing "is that usually people are not completely healed by prayer, but they are improved."[3] He believes that "prayer for healing is often a process. It requires time."[4] Whereas minor ailments may be healed quickly through prayer, it is "the long term organic problems, such as a broken bone, or a palpable tumor, that take the most time."[5]

Marilyn Hickey appeals to this notion of gradual or progressive healing to explain why people are prayed for with no apparent change.

> Remember that God's Word is like seed planted in one's spirit. When we plant carrot seeds, we don't run out and pull carrots the next day! We plant the seed of God's Word in faith, believing that by His stripes we were healed. We must water that seed every day by confessing and believing God's Word. The day will come when the healing will become evident, because the seeds will have matured. Sometimes people plant these "seeds" at an advanced stage of illness, so it takes more time for the life of God's Word to manifest. That is why it is important to plant God's Word in our hearts before Satan ever tries to attack us with sickness. Then the roots of sickness and disease will have no place in our lives.[6]

While we may rightly speak of God's Word as a seed planted in one's spirit, there is no biblical justification for applying this analogy to bodily healing. Where in the New Testament is *healing* ever described as a seed planted in the spirit, which only after a considerable period of time becomes evident to us? Where in the New Testament are we told that the power of God's Word is hindered by the "advanced stage" of an illness? We certainly never see anything remotely approaching this in the healing ministry of Jesus.

John Wimber acknowledges that "most of the healings in the New Testament were immediate, though not all."[7] Which ones were not immediate? Wimber gives only *one* example, the healing of the blind man at Bethsaida (Mark 8:22-26). He then concludes that "most physical healing is a process, because sometimes there are other factors—emotional, psychological, demonic—that must first be dealt with."[8] This logic escapes me. If "most" (according to Wimber, *all but one*) healings in the New Testament were immediate, why are "most" healings today progressive? These "other factors" which Wimber mentions (emotional, psychological, demonic) were just as real and operative in the first century as they are now, yet they posed no problem for Jesus.

It will not do to say, "Well, that was Jesus, and we are only sinful men." Remember, the charismatic always insists that it is *Jesus*, not he or she, who heals today. And Jesus is the same yesterday, today, and forever. And Jesus loves us as much today as he loved people back then. And miracles are as much God's will and way for the church in the twentieth century as in the first. If the charismatic believes all these things, and he does, he is hard-pressed to explain why we so rarely see instantaneous and total healing of *all* kinds of diseases as was the case in the first century.

Michael Harper is yet another charismatic author who wrestles with this problem. Here is his explanation.

> Sometimes it has been argued that Jesus' healings were so complete that there was never any need for convalescence afterwards. This has been used as evidence that Jesus' healing ministry was unique and not to be compared with the modern healing movement in which a period of convalescence is usually

required. But such comparisons are misleading. In the first place we are simply not told what happened afterwards to many of those whom Jesus healed. Some may have needed convalescence, others may have experienced gradual healing. Some modern healings through faith in Jesus Christ have in my experience needed no convalescence and been instantaneous [Harper here gives one example]. . . . It is true that some instances of modern healing are gradual. But it is jumping to conclusions to surmise that all Jesus' healings were like this one [he is referring to the healing of Peter's mother-in-law in Luke 4:38-39]. There is no clear evidence since the followup to most of them is not documented.[9]

Here we find Harper basing his entire position not on what the Bible explicitly says, but on what it does *not* say. He speculates concerning what *might* have happened to people Jesus healed about whom the Bible says nothing more. But on what basis does he speculate in this way? Is it on the basis of *anything* the Bible says about the nature of Jesus' healing ministry or about the people whom Jesus healed? No. Clearly, Harper bases his speculation on what he has found to be true in the contemporary healing movement. He reasons like this: Since most *today* are not immediately healed, it must be that many in the first century were not immediately healed. He says this even though all the biblical evidence is to the contrary. It is not an ill-founded or premature conclusion to surmise that all Jesus' healings were like his healing of Peter's mother-in-law. That conclusion is based on what the Bible explicitly says concerning the people whom Jesus *did* heal, and about whom information is provided subsequent to their encounter with the Savior.

Is there any indication in Scripture that the people Jesus healed were not healed immediately or totally? Charismatics often point to three passages they believe provide exceptions to the general rule. The first is Luke 17:11-19 and the case of the ten lepers. When Jesus "saw them, He said to them, 'Go and show yourselves to the priests.' And it came about that as they were going, they were cleansed" (Luke 17:14).

But notice three important facts concerning this incident. First, the text nowhere says that Jesus began to heal or cleanse the lepers upon his initial encounter with them. It does not say, "Jesus touched them, but only later as they were on their way, they were healed." All that Jesus did was to instruct them, in accordance with Levitical law, to go and show themselves to the priests. Not until they were going, did Jesus heal them of their disease. Second, the reason for not healing them until they were on their way may well have been to provide an occasion to highlight the gratitude of the one (a Samaritan), as over against the ingratitude of the remaining nine. Jesus himself made this clear when he said to the one grateful man: "Were there not ten cleansed? But the nine—where are they? Were none found who turned back to give glory to God, except this foreigner?" (Luke 17:17-18). Finally, notice that when Jesus *did* heal them, he healed them wholly. There is no indication in the passage of a *partial* healing followed by a *complete* one. There was no period of convalescence, but an immediate and radical disappearance of all trace of the disease.

Some also appeal to John 9 as an exceptional case. But again, there was no partial or gradual healing of the blind man followed by a complete restoration of his sight. The reason he received his sight after washing in the pool of Siloam is that only then had he obeyed Jesus' instructions (John 9:6-7). Jesus obviously did not intend for him to be healed *until* then. When he had done what Jesus had said, the man's sight was instantaneously and wholly restored.

But what about the blind man in Mark 8:22-26? We read:

> And taking the blind man by the hand, He brought him out of the village; and after spitting in his eyes, and laying His hands upon him, He asked him, "Do you see anything?" And he looked up and said, "I see men, for I am seeing them like trees walking about." Then again He laid His hands upon his eyes; and he looked intently and was restored, and began to see everything clearly (Mark 8:23-25).

The event described here is unusual. For example, it is only one of two healings (the other is Mark 7:31-37) recorded in Mark alone. It is also the only healing in which Jesus asks the individual if his action has been effective ("Do you see anything?"). Furthermore, this is the only healing in which Jesus lays hands on the individual twice. And it is the only healing in all of the Gospels in which a partial recovery precedes a full recovery. What makes this even more exceptional is that Mark's Gospel is known for its emphasis on the immediacy of Christ's healings (see Mark 1:42; 2:12; 5:29, 42; 10:52).

So why is this one healing a gradual one? In the first place, "gradual" or "progressive" are hardly appropriate terms to describe a healing that was *complete* within a matter of seconds. Unlike a situation where total healing comes days or even weeks following an initial encounter, this man had his sight fully restored to him presently. His experience bears little in common with the "progressive" or "gradual" healings many claim today, in which days, weeks, even months pass, often with no full recovery. Efforts to make this exceptional incident the norm for all healings indicate the shaky theological ground on which many faith healers stand.

So why did Jesus heal the man in two stages, even if the stages were separated by only seconds? We don't know. There is not the slightest hint in this text that the man lacked sufficient faith. And let's not forget that he was wholly healed only moments after Jesus first touched him. If his faith was weak, it wasn't weak for long! Neither is it likely that his healing was in two stages because of the severity of his blindness. Commentators are in general agreement that this man did not suffer from congenital blindness. After all, he knew what trees and men looked like (Mark 8:24). But even if he was blind from birth, that would present no obstacle for a healer who had already proved he could raise people from the dead!

John Calvin has suggested that Jesus deliberately broke with his normal pattern for healing in order to remind his disciples of his sovereign freedom to heal whenever and however he pleased. In other words, it "was probably done to set up in the man a proof of his [Christ's] freedom of activity, that He was not tied to any rigid form; but exercised his power in this way or that. . . . Thus the grace of Christ which on others was poured out all at once, flowed upon this man drop by drop."[10] Beyond this we can only speculate.

ADDENDUM
THE MEANING OF JOHN 14:12

In his discourse in the upper room Jesus told his disciples, "Truly, truly I say to you, he who believes in Me, the works that I do shall he do also; and greater works than these shall he do; because I go to the Father" (John 14:12). If one thinks about the "works" Jesus performed, such as calming the sea of Galilee, feeding the five thousand, and raising Lazarus from the dead, this promise in John 14:12 quickly captures the attention. The suggestion, however, that we might somehow do greater miracles than Jesus has not set well with everyone. Some seek to evade this interpretation by arguing that the promise had relevance only to Jesus' immediate listeners. That is, the apostolic company alone, during the apostolic age, may reasonably expect to do greater works than Jesus (cf. 2 Cor. 12:12; Heb. 2:4).

The problem with restricting this promise to the apostles is that Jesus spoke in unrestricted terms. The only qualification he placed on this promise is that one must believe in him. "He who believes in Me" is our Lord's way of describing any Christian. All believers, he appears to say, shall do greater works than I. So what may we as Christians, as men and women who believe in him, justifiably expect as we go forth to minister the gospel?

It seems to me that the first thing we must do in order to understand this passage is to examine the book of Acts. After all, Acts is the record of the "works" or "acts" performed by those present with Jesus on the night he uttered the words in question.

There is no denying that the apostles performed miracles by the power of God. The narrative in Acts makes that clear (see the next chapter). But were the miracles they performed greater or more numerous than the ones Jesus performed? Were they more sensational? The answer to both questions is no. Nowhere do we read in Acts or anywhere else in the New Testament that the first century disciples of Jesus healed the multitudes with greater success than he did. There were no miracles of creation in Acts, such as multiplying a few loaves of bread and fish into enough food to feed thousands of people. Instead, we read in Acts 11:27-30 of a great famine that struck during the reign of Claudius. "And in the proportion that any of the disciples had means, each of them determined to send a contribution for the relief of the brethren living in Judea. And this they did, sending it in charge of Barnabas and Saul to the elders" (Acts 11:29-30). But surely if John 14:12 means what many charismatics today say it means, the apostles would not have found it necessary to collect money to send to the believers in Judea who were suffering for lack of food. If they were promised by Jesus himself that they would do greater works than he, a prayer meeting over a basket of leftovers would have sufficed to alleviate the problem. Yet we read that even Saul (Paul), perhaps the greatest of the apostolic miracle-workers, rather than multiplying food for the hungry, took an active role in conveying funds to the afflicted brethren.

Turning water into wine was the first of Jesus' public miracles, yet we read of nothing remotely approaching this deed in the ministry of the apostles. Nor do we read of their calming the sea or walking upon it, although that would surely have been an effective evangelistic device for the apostle Paul when he suffered shipwreck in Acts 27. The apostles never maneuvered fish into nets or paid their taxes with money found in the mouth of one of them. We simply do not see miracles in the book of Acts that are equivalent to, much less "greater than," those performed by Jesus. But why not, if Jesus really meant in John 14:12 what we are told he meant? Why are there hospitals and cemeteries and famines and fishing wars and hurricanes? If faith in Jesus is the only requirement to perform miracles greater than the ones he performed, why don't Christians ban together in prayer to put an immediate end to the cause of so much woe and suffering and heartache in this world?

The answer is not that Jesus promised us something he has failed to fulfill. Perhaps we have misunderstood what he meant when he spoke of works "greater" than his own. We need to ask ourselves this question: In what sense are the works the church performs "greater" than the ones Jesus did, and what accounts for their greatness? The answer to the second half of that question is not hard to come by. Jesus tells us in the closing words of John 14:12: we will do greater works than Jesus *because he is going to the Father.*

The significance of Christ's ascension and exaltation is seen principally in the coming of the Holy Spirit. That much is clear from
John 14:16-17 and John 16:7-11. Evidently the consummation of
Christ's redemptive work secured for his followers an even more
powerful ministry of the Spirit than Jesus himself experienced
while on the earth. But if that is true, in what way or ways have we
done works greater than those of our Lord?

If we look again at the book of Acts we discover that there is
really only one area in which the early church exceeded the Lord
Jesus. There is only one "work" of the church that may justifiably
be called "greater" than that which Jesus did. I am referring, of
course, to the salvation of lost souls. Not that the apostles were
better evangelists than Jesus was. But the power and presence of
the Spirit available to them (and to us) following Pentecost made
possible a greater harvest of souls than anything our Lord saw during his earthly sojourn. Jesus himself prophesied of this before his
ascension. He told his followers that when the Holy Spirit would
come, they would be endued with a power that would enable them
to take the gospel far beyond the bounds of Christ's own ministry.
They would see the lost saved not only in Jerusalem but also "in all
Judea and Samaria, and even the remotest part of the earth" (Acts
1:8). This would occur only after the Holy Spirit had come in consequence of Christ's ascension to the right hand of the Father
(John 14:12). On the day of Pentecost alone, because of the presence and power of the Spirit, more people were saved through the
preaching of Peter than were saved through the preaching of Jesus
during his entire three-year public ministry (cf. Acts 2:41, 47).

So we see that the early church did indeed do the works of Jesus:
they healed the sick, cast out evil spirits, and even on occasion
raised the dead. But the one work that was truly "greater" than
that of Jesus, in terms of both quality (because it involved more
than the physical and bodily) and quantity, was the expansion of
the church through the salvation of lost souls.

Finally, we may also find help in determining the meaning of
John 14:12 by looking at a similar statement in Matthew 11:11. There
Jesus said, "Truly I say to you, among those born of women there
has not arisen anyone greater than John the Baptist; yet he who is

least in the kingdom of heaven is greater than he." John was obviously a great man. His role in the ministry of Jesus was of such importance that his birth was described in great detail by Luke (Luke 1:5-25, 57-80), in conjunction with Luke's equally detailed description of the birth of Jesus himself (Luke 1:26-56; 2:1-20). It was John who "came for a witness, that he might bear witness of the light, that all might believe through him. He was not the light, but came that he might bear witness of the light" (John 1:7-8). Notwithstanding John's greatness, "he who is least in the kingdom of heaven is greater than he." But how can this be?

It would appear that although John was great, he never experienced during his earthly life the fullness of the blessings of the kingdom of heaven, which came through the death and especially the resurrection of Jesus (the same, of course, is true of all Old Testament saints; cf. Hebrews 11:39-40). John's ministry came too early in redemptive history to permit him to participate in the glory of the new age, which Jesus inaugurated. He was truly the greatest of the prophets (Matt. 11:7-10), says D. A. Carson, "because he pointed most unambiguously to Jesus. Nevertheless even the least in the kingdom is greater yet because, living after the crucial revelatory and eschatological events have occurred, he or she points to Jesus still more unambiguously than John the Baptist."[11]

Carson believes that something similar to this may stand behind our Lord's words in John 14:12, and I am inclined to agree with him. When Jesus says that his going to the Father will lead to "greater works" on the part of his followers, he indicates that a new day in the history of redemption is about to dawn. It is a day, an age, in which the disciples will experience something not even Jesus experienced. Carson explains:

> His work brought it about: but then he left and did not himself participate in it (in his bodily presence) after Pentecost. This does not mean that Jesus' disciples are greater than he is. It does mean that their works are greater than his in this respect, that they are privileged to participate in the effects of Jesus' completed work. Until he returned to his Father and bestowed the Holy Spirit, everything Jesus did was of neces-

sity still incomplete. By contrast, the works of the disciples participate in the new situation that exists once Jesus' work is complete. Their works are greater in that they are privileged to take place after the moment of fulfillment.[12]

9

HEALING IN THE BOOK OF ACTS

Not long ago I had the opportunity to hear Dr. Adrian Rogers, past president of the Southern Baptist Convention and pastor of Bellvue Baptist Church in Memphis, Tennessee, preach a series of sermons on the book of Acts. The title of the series was "Give Me That Old-Time Religion!" Many of us would like nothing more than to see that old-time religion we read about in Acts make an appearance in our own day. The church of Jesus Christ in the twentieth century could certainly profit from the infectious zeal and self-sacrifice so prominent among first-century believers. There was a quality of commitment and conviction in those men and women that is all too rare in the church today. Although many things may be said about Christians in the last quarter of the twentieth century, few of us have been accused of turning "the world upside down" (Acts 17:6, KJV)!

But to what extent should we really desire or expect to see church life in the first century repeated in the twentieth? Is everything that happened then relevant and applicable now? Students of the Bible are divided on this point. Some believe that "if it was good enough for Peter, it's good enough for me!" Others insist that much of what we see in Acts was temporary and transitional. God's purpose for us, they say, may very well differ in significant respects from his purpose for the early church.

That is a huge question with many major implications—too many to address in this book. But one issue does concern us here, the reality of divine healing in the narrative of Acts. Several instances need to be carefully examined to determine their relevance for our expectations concerning healing in the contemporary church.

Acts 3:1-4:12 (cf. Acts 8:4-8; 9:32-35)

When Peter stood to preach on the day of Pentecost, he rebuked the leaders of Israel for having rejected Jesus, "a man attested to you by God with miracles and wonders and signs which God performed through Him in your midst" (2:22). Although Jesus was himself no longer on the earth, the "miracles" God performed through him were still operative among his disciples. Luke says of the early church that "everyone kept feeling a sense of awe; and many wonders and signs were taking place through the apostles" (2:43). Offering a vivid illustration, Luke goes on to describe in great detail one particular healing. It is the story of a man "who had been lame from his mother's womb" (3:2). This incident and its implications take up all of chapter 3 and over half of chapter 4. Several things about this healing merit our consideration.

First, this man bears no resemblance to the sort of people usually seen at modern healing services. Crutches were useless to him. To get anywhere he had to be "carried" along (3:2) and set down by his friends. He didn't suffer from arthritis or a sprained ankle or a broken leg. He was congenitally lame. I'm not suggesting that those who make their way to the front of a healing line today are not suffering. They are often in considerable discomfort. One may have strained his back while moving furniture; another may have an arthritic elbow. But these kinds of infirmities do not compare with the man in Acts 3. His affliction would not in time heal itself. No amount of emotional hype or manipulative organ music would have had any effect on him. For 40 years (Acts 4:22) he had been without any use of his legs. His was not a gradual restoration from partial impairment to complete mobility. He was healed instantaneously and wholly (cf. Acts 9:32-35). There was no period of recuperation or convalescence. We are told that when Peter seized him by the right hand and raised him up: "immediately his feet and ankles were strengthened. And with a leap, he stood upright and began to walk; and he entered the temple with them, walking and leaping and praising God" (3:7-8).

A second important factor is that this healing was public so that there might be no doubt about what had happened. It was a visible, empirically verifiable healing. Luke says that "all the people saw him walking and praising God; and they were taking note of him as being the one who used to sit at the Beautiful Gate of the temple to beg alms, and they were filled with wonder and amazement at what had happened to him" (3:9-10). The healing was so unmistakable and beyond dispute that even unbelievers were forced to concede its reality. When the rulers and elders and scribes of Israel, among which were Annas the high priest, Caiaphas, John, and Alexander (4:5-6), saw the man who had been healed, "they had nothing to say in reply" (4:14)! Conferring secretly, they said to one another: "What shall we do with these men? For the fact that a noteworthy miracle has taken place through them is apparent to all who live in Jerusalem, and we cannot deny it. But in order that it may not spread any further among the people, let us warn them to speak no more to any man in this name" (4:16-17). (Note that notwithstanding their confession that the "miracle" really occurred, they remained in unbelief [cf. Luke 16:19-31].)

Third, Peter makes it clear that the source of the healing was divine. It was not by any "power" or "piety" in the apostles themselves (3:12), but "by the name of Jesus Christ, the Nazarene . . . [that] this man stands here . . . in good health" (4:10).

Finally, the role of faith is important in this case. Peter says that it is "the name of Jesus which has strengthened this man whom you see and know; and the faith which comes through Him has given him this perfect health in the presence of you all" (3:16). Unfortunately Peter does not tell us whose faith he is describing, or even what the content of that faith might be. Was it the faith of Peter and John that led to the healing? Perhaps their steadfast belief in the authority and power of Jesus over illness is in view. Or again it may well be the faith of the man himself, although nowhere in chapters 3 and 4 is faith ever explicitly attributed to him. If it was his faith, what did he believe, and in whom or what had he placed his faith? Again, we cannot be certain.

In all likelihood, though, it was *saving* faith in Jesus and those truths concerning him which Peter later proclaimed in his sermon. That is to say, this man's body was healed at the same time his soul was saved, when he placed his faith in the Jesus who was "delivered up and disowned in the presence of Pilate" (3:13), the Jesus who was put to death, "whom God raised from the dead" (3:15).

Nowhere does Peter so much as hint that this man was healed because he believed that God could and *would* heal him. Peter didn't tell him to deny his symptoms though they remained unchanged. He didn't command him to claim his healing or to rid his mind of all doubt concerning God's will in the matter. If the "faith" Peter mentions was that of the man himself, there is no reason to think it was anything other than the faith you and I exercise by God's grace when we turn to Christ for the forgiveness of our sins.

Let me state clearly that I would be thrilled should God decide to heal the congenitally lame today as he did on that day so many centuries ago. And I do not doubt for a moment that he is perfectly capable of doing so. If he should choose to heal in this fashion, his purpose would be to bring glory and honor to his own name (4:21). But I am deeply disturbed by the claims being made for so-called "miraculous healings" today that do not even remotely compare with the healing of this man in Acts 3-4. If modern faith healers wish to use Acts 3-4 as an example and precedent for their own ministries, let them in the name of Jesus heal those who haven't taken a step from birth. If Jesus wills to heal today no less than he did then, and if the authority and power to do so are as available to us as to Peter and John, then come with me to Children's Hospital in Oklahoma City in order that those precious little children whose bodies are twisted and deformed may be spared the 40 years of anguish this man in Acts endured.

Acts 5:12-16

In a much briefer statement Luke tells us that what happened in Acts 3-4 was no isolated incident in the early church. Unlike many in healing ministries today whose success is sporadic and uncertain, the apostles healed *all* who came to them (5:16).

One verse in particular is especially interesting. In Acts 5:15 Luke says that the sick were being placed on cots and pallets in the street "so that when Peter came by, at least his shadow might fall on any one of them." If indeed people were healed when Peter's shadow fell upon them, it was not because of any magical power in the shadow itself. The shadow was simply a way of making contact with the man whom God had empowered with the authority to heal.

However, we cannot be certain that people were actually healed in this way. Luke does refer to people being healed in verse 16, but not in verse 15. It may well be that in verse 15 he is merely recording what these people believed about Peter's shadow, without himself endorsing the idea. We know that in many primitive cultures, and even sporadically in the Mediterranean countries in the first century, a man's shadow was thought to be equivalent to his soul or to the vital part of his personality. People believed it was dangerous to let one's shadow fall upon a particular person or object. Many even feared midday, because that is when one's shadow virtually disappears.[1] In Acts 5:15 Luke may be alluding to this belief, without implying that he himself believes it or that any are actually healed in that way. We simply don't know for sure.

Acts 9:36-43; 20:7-12

There are only two cases of actual bodily resurrection from the dead recorded in Acts. In the first incident, a woman named Tabitha fell sick and died. But she was not just any woman. She is specifically described by Luke as a woman "abounding with deeds of kindness and charity, which she continually did" (9:36). If the charismatics are correct concerning the relation between sin and sickness, why did she get sick, and why was it fatal? It seems as if Luke is trying to tell us something when he describes her godly virtue and immediately follows that with, "and it came about *at that time* that she fell sick and died" (9:37). Not only was it not because she had sinned; it was *in spite of the fact* that she was saintly that she fell sick and died!

The second account of a resurrection from the dead is provided in Acts 20:7-12. As a preacher I am encouraged by this story, if only because it indicates that I'm not the only one who puts people to sleep! Even the great apostle Paul was up to the task. (But then again, my preaching never killed anyone either. At least, not that I'm aware of.)

This is the case of young Eutyches who evidently fell prey to the soothing aroma and heat generated by the "many lamps" (20:8) being used. His tragic and fatal fall resulted in an expression of divine power through the apostle Paul, who embraced the young boy and restored him to life.

Acts 10:38

Peter says in Acts 10:38 that Jesus' earthly ministry entailed "healing all who were oppressed by the devil." Although this does not say anything directly about healing in the early church, it raises the important question of the relationship between the devil and disease. We know from the Gospels that Satan was occasionally the source of sickness (cf. Luke 8:1-2; 13:11-17; Matt. 9:32-33; and perhaps Matt. 8:16). But in the great majority of cases there is no reference to the devil or other evil spirits as the immediate and direct cause of bodily illness. In light of this fact, some charismatics are more cautious than others in attributing disease to the devil. John Wimber, for example, says that "not *all* cases of disease are caused by demons or are demons. Often, of course, there are psychological or physical explanations for illness. But more frequently than many Western Christians realize, the cause is demonic."[2]

Others, however, who are more prone to put the blame on Satan often use Acts 10:38 to make their point. T. J. McCrossan insists that Acts 10:38 "proves to us conclusively that all the diseases Christ cured while on earth had been caused by Satan."[3] In another place he argues that "every sickness, disease, and deformity Christ cured while on earth was the result of Satan's work, and *it is the same today*."[4] According to Kenneth Hagin, Acts 10:38 says "that every one of these sick persons Jesus healed was oppressed of the devil. And do you notice what the Bible calls sickness? Satanic oppression."[5]

But of course Acts 10:38 says no such thing. The passage says that everyone who was oppressed of the devil was healed by Jesus. That is not the same thing as saying that if someone needed healing, it was always because of Satanic oppression. McCrossan and Hagin have made a fundamental logical error in their attempt to read a preconceived theology into this text. Let me illustrate. Suppose I were to say, "Dr. Jones was a compassionate physician who treated all who suffered from athlete's foot." It would be wrong to conclude from this that *everyone* Dr. Jones treated had athlete's foot! He may also have had patients who suffered from tonsillitis or ulcers or measles, and so on. In short, the statement "All athlete's foot sufferers were treated" would not imply the conclusion "All who were treated were athlete's foot sufferers."

Likewise Peter's statement that all the demonically oppressed were healed by Jesus does not mean that all who were healed were demonically oppressed. In fact, as we can readily see from reading the four Gospels, very few of those whom Jesus healed are said to have suffered because of demonic oppression.

Is it possible that some people today become ill because of demonic influence? Yes, that is certainly a possibility. But in view of what the New Testament says concerning the defeat of Satan by our Lord's death, resurrection, and exaltation, I am persuaded that the devil and demons have far less to do with bodily illness now, subsequent to Christ's work, than they did before it. (For more on this, see Appendix A, "The Defeat of the Devil.")

Acts 14:8-10 (cf. 28:7-10)

We find in Acts 14:8-10 a healing identical to the one described in Acts 3-4, except that in this case it is Paul, not Peter, through whom the Lord heals. Both cases, however, involve a man "lame from his mother's womb, who had never walked" (14:8). And in both cases faith plays a decisive role in the healing. Unlike the story in Acts 3-4, here the faith referred to is clearly that of the man being healed (cf. v. 9). The only information Luke provides us is that "he had faith to be made well" (v. 9). In view of what we have already seen in the Gospels and elsewhere, his faith probably consisted of an unswerving confidence in the power of the Christ whom Paul preached. Recognizing this, Paul "said with a loud voice, 'Stand upright on your feet.' And he leaped up and began to walk" (v. 10). Although no one can be dogmatic about the precise content of this man's faith, of this we may be sure: he was healed *immediately* and *wholly* of a *congenital* affliction.

Acts 19:11-12

The description of Paul's healing power in Acts 19:11-12 is reminiscent of Mark 5:25-28 (and perhaps Acts 5:15). In that passage the woman who had suffered from a hemorrhage for 12 years was persuaded that if she could but touch Jesus' garments she would be healed. And that is precisely what happened. Jesus himself is described as having perceived that "the power proceeding from Him had gone forth" (5:30). Evidently God had endowed the apostle Paul with a similar power to heal. For we read in this passage that "God was performing extraordinary miracles by the hands of Paul, so that handkerchiefs or aprons were even carried from his body to the sick, and the diseases left them and the evil spirits went out" (19:11-12). The "handkerchiefs" had probably been used by Paul as headbands to absorb perspiration as he worked. The "aprons" no doubt were used to protect his clothing.

It has been suggested that this approach to healing differs very little from some of the methods employed by Jesus. We are reminded that Jesus used saliva (Mark 7:31-37) and clay (John 9:6) in the healing of the sick. However, in both of these instances Jesus was physically present when the healing occurred. Paul, according to Acts 19, was absent, and that has led many to conclude that God somehow infused these material objects with healing power. The text, however, says no such thing. All that we may conclude from the passage is that when these handkerchiefs and aprons were taken from Paul to the sick, God healed them. The power was in God, not the material objects.

Undoubtedly many are uneasy with this passage in Acts because of outlandish attempts by certain faith healers to repeat the practice in our day. Often, unlike Paul, they charge a substantial fee for their "prayer cloths" and "anointed aprons." Such an abuse of the biblical practice should not diminish our appreciation of what God did through Paul. But we are left with the question, Why did God choose to operate through Paul in this fashion?

Unfortunately, Luke does not tell us, and so we must not be dogmatic in trying to answer the question. One reason may have been the logistical impossibility of Paul's ministering directly to each and every sick person. Paul was not omnipresent! These handkerchiefs and aprons, therefore, compensated for his absence. It is also likely that this method was selected precisely because it was unusual and thus was well suited to confirm and solidify the authenticity of the message Paul proclaimed, as well as his own authority as an apostle (cf. 2 Cor. 12:12). Since *only* Paul is said to have employed this means, it may well be that God intended it exclusively for him as a witness to the veracity of his claims.

Two other factors lead me to believe that this was a unique healing phenomenon, not normative for others either in Paul's day or our own. First, we should remember that Paul was in *Ephesus* when these incidents occurred (cf. 19:1ff.). Ephesus had a reputation as a center for the magical arts (cf. Acts 19:18-19). It was the home for numerous cults and superstitious practices, particularly the worship of Artemis (Latin, Diana), "the multibreasted goddess of fertility,"[6] whose temple in Ephesus was one of the Seven Wonders of the ancient world. It is entirely possible, therefore, that the use of handkerchiefs and aprons as media for divine healing (if that is in fact what they were) was God's way of accommodating to the religious mindset of the city's inhabitants. By meeting these people on their own cultural grounds Paul was better equipped to communicate the truth of Christ. In any other context such a method for divine healing would have been singularly inappropriate. But conditions in Ephesus may supply an explanation for the peculiar method of healing in this passage.

Second, and related to the above factor, we are told in verse 11 that God performed "extraordinary miracles" through Paul. What makes this language noteworthy is that a miracle is by definition something out of the ordinary. So why does Luke describe Paul's miracles as "extraordinary"? The Greek phrase translated "extraordinary" in our English versions is never used in other passages to describe a miracle, whether healing or otherwise. In fact, it occurs only one other time in Acts (28:2), in reference to the "extraordinary kindness" shown to Paul by the natives of Malta.

In other words, there are miracles, and then there is what God did through Paul in Ephesus—an extraordinary display of divine healing for which there is neither a biblical precedent nor a repeat occurrence. Since in the inspired record it happened only once, is there biblical warrant for us to expect healing through "prayer cloths" and the like today?

We may broaden that question in the light of our brief survey of healing in the book of Acts. Comparing contemporary claims for miraculous healing with what we find in God's Word, is what we see happening today the same as happened back then? What, therefore, may or may not we *expect* in regard to miraculous healing in our time?

10

HEALING IN THE EPISTLES

Most people are convinced that, comparatively speaking, the New Testament epistles tell us little about divine healing. Certainly, there are fewer references to healing in the epistles than in the Gospels and the book of Acts. But what the epistles *do* say on this subject, though little, is of immense importance. In fact, it is so important that I am devoting three chapters to it. Two passages, 2 Corinthians 12:7-10, and James 5:13-16, deserve chapters of their own. In this chapter we will take a long look at several other passages, all but one of which were written by the apostle Paul.

Romans 8:11
Here Paul says that "if the Spirit of Him who raised Jesus from the dead dwells in you, He who raised Christ Jesus from the dead will also give life to your mortal bodies through His Spirit who indwells you" (Rom. 8:11). Surprisingly, charismatics appeal to this verse to support their view on miraculous healing. They insist that the phrase "give life to your mortal bodies" refers not only to bodily resurrection in the future, but also (if not primarily) to bodily healing in the present.[1] There are several problems with this interpretation.

In the first place, it is utterly foreign to the context. Nowhere in Romans 8, either before or after this passage, does Paul say anything about divine healing. The only thing remotely approaching a discussion of the body is in verses 18-25, where Paul asserts that *suffering* is precisely what all Christians may *expect* in this life until the final redemption of the body at Christ's return (cf. v. 23).

The charismatic interpretation also encounters a problem with verse 10, where Paul says that "if Christ is in you, though the body

is dead because of sin, yet the spirit is alive because of righteousness." His point is that the body is subject to decay, deterioration,
and eventual death because of sin. Nevertheless, we should rejoice,
for though the body must die physically, the presence of the Holy
Spirit is the guarantee of resurrection life. In other words, verse 10
is the answer to Paul's desperate cry of Romans 7:24: "Wretched
man that I am! Who will set me free from the body of this death?"

Another problem with finding bodily healing in this passage is
the explicit reference to the resurrection of Christ from the dead.
Paul is saying that since the Spirit of Him [i.e., God the Father]
who raised Jesus from the dead is in you, rest assured that he will
do for you what he did for Jesus, namely, *raise you bodily from the
dead.* The reality of *Christ's bodily resurrection* is the foundation of
the hope and certainty of *ours.* In other words, Paul is concerned
with bodily resurrection, not bodily healing.

Finally, the word Paul uses here that is translated "give life" or
"quicken" (KJV) is found 11 times in the New Testament. In every
case it refers either to the giving of spiritual life in regeneration (the
new birth) or to the giving of physical life in bodily resurrection.
Nowhere does it carry the meaning "to heal" or "to accelerate the
life processes of our physical bodies."[2] I can only conclude that
Romans 8:11 provides no support for the belief that the ministry of
the Holy Spirit guarantees or even provides the reasonable expectation of bodily healing in this life.

The Word of Knowledge (1 Cor. 12:8)

The first time I saw this spiritual gift allegedly in operation was
on the 700 Club several years ago. As Pat Robertson and co-host
Ben Kinchlow were praying, they both suddenly began to speak as
if God the Holy Spirit were imparting information to them concerning the bodily affliction of men and women of whom they had
no prior knowledge. "There is a young man in Texas," Robertson
might say, "who is suffering from kidney stones. God is healing you
right now. Praise Jesus!" I soon came to discover that charismatic
Christians identified this experience with the "word of knowledge,"
one of the many spiritual gifts mentioned by Paul in 1 Corinthians

12. There the apostle says that "to each one is given the manifestation of the Spirit for the common good. For to one is given the word of wisdom through the Spirit, and to another the word of knowledge according to the same Spirit."

John Wimber defines a word of knowledge as: "God revealing facts about a situation concerning which a person had no previous knowledge. An example of this is God giving someone exact details of a person's life, to reveal sin, warn and provide safety, reveal thoughts, provide healing or provide instructions."[3] Wimber gives one illustration of a word of knowledge that he experienced while on an airplane. He claims that he saw the word "ADULTERY" across a man's forehead. "I was seeing it not with my eyes," says Wimber, "but in my mind's eye. No one else on the plane, I am sure, saw it."[4] (Wimber goes on to relate how he confronted the man, who then confessed to his infidelity and repented.)

Although charismatics such as Wimber contend that a word of knowledge may prove helpful in all kinds of settings,[5] it is most frequently operative when divine healing occurs. In fact, it functions almost as a precondition for healing, without which it is difficult to minister successfully to those who are afflicted. For example, Michael Harper says this of the word of knowledge:

> It is of the utmost importance that we have a revelation from God [i.e., a word of knowledge] concerning every possible aspect of human sickness. Is it due to human sin, and are there particular sins which need to be confessed? Are there demonic forces involved, and what are they? What mental attitudes are there which may be blocking healing? Is it God's will to heal instantly or later? Are other people involved?[6]

According to Harper, the Holy Spirit answers these questions by direct divine revelation in order to facilitate the healing experience. "We need to know," says Harper, "what really lies behind every kind of sickness."[7]

The means by which the Spirit conveys this information are varied. "Sometimes," explains Wimber, "I receive a pain in a part of my body that parallels the ailment in someone else God wants to heal. Other times I have a flash of intuition about someone."[8] On occasion such divine insights "come as impressions: specific words, pictures in my mind's eye, physical sensations in my body that correspond to problems in their bodies."[9]

Michael Harper, among others, insists that Jesus himself had the gift of the word of knowledge.

> Again and again he was able to see things which were hidden from most people. He called complete strangers by name. He said to the man lowered through the roof that his sins were forgiven, when he had been brought to Jesus for healing. Jesus was able to see the whole situation, and make decisions on the basis of knowledge and information he could only have received from the Holy Spirit. At the pool of Bethesda he knew all about the one man he healed. He could read people like a book.[10]

Indeed Jesus "could read people like a book." But there is no indication that he was blessed with the *spiritual gift* Paul describes in 1 Corinthians 12. Whereas Jesus healed the sick and prophesied, there is no evidence that he did so by virtue of a *charisma*, a spiritual gift, such as we read about in the epistles. Spiritual gifts are manifestations of the Spirit granted to the church subsequent to Pentecost. They are designed for the edification of the body of Christ. It is anachronistic, therefore, to identify displays of divine power in Jesus' ministry with those gifts which come to the church after Jesus was exalted. Furthermore, the knowledge and insight Jesus had of people and circumstances were far more likely due to his *deity*. He knew what men were thinking, what they had done, their needs, and their desires not because he had the gift of the word of knowledge, but because he was God!

The word of knowledge and the word of wisdom are nowhere mentioned in the New Testament outside of 1 Corinthians 12:8. Nothing there would lead us to believe that these gifts were possessed and practiced by Jesus. Nor is there evidence that the word of knowledge has anything to do with healing or divinely imparted information concerning the cause or nature of an illness. Nothing in Scripture would lead us to expect to see words like "adultery" (or "thievery" or "jealousy") emblazoned across someone's forehead. It is one thing for people today to claim to have such experiences. It is something else entirely for them to identify those experiences with the spiritual gift of the word of knowledge.

What, then, did Paul mean when he spoke of the word of wisdom and the word of knowledge? Notice first of all, that these two gifts are omitted from the other listings of the charismata in the New Testament (cf. Rom. 12; Eph. 4; 1 Pet. 4). Might there have been something distinctive in *Corinth* itself that accounts for Paul's reference to these two gifts? I believe the answer is yes. Ralph Martin reminds us that "wisdom" and "knowledge" were "clearly watchwords among the people there, especially as the church lay under the spell of an incipient Gnosticism that set great store by these qualities."[11] James Dunn refers to these two terms as "slogans of the faction opposing Paul in Corinth."[12] In fact, it was because his opponents claimed to possess a special "wisdom" and a special "knowledge" others did not have that Paul felt compelled to discuss these concepts at length. According to Dunn, "This is why *gnōsis* [knowledge] keeps recurring within the Corinthian letters and only rarely elsewhere, and why 1 Cor. 1-3 is so dominated by discussion of *sophia* [wisdom]."[13]

When one finally realizes that it was "in the name of wisdom [that] the Corinthians were rejecting both Paul and his gospel,"[14] it comes as little surprise that he would say so much about it. Consider these comments from 1 Corinthians 1.

For the word of the cross is to those who are perishing foolishness, but to us who are being saved it is the power of God. For it is written, "I will destroy the *wisdom* of the *wise*, and the cleverness of the clever I will set aside." Where is the *wise* man? Where is the scribe? Where is the debater of this age? Has not God made foolish *the wisdom of the world*? For since in the *wisdom* of God *the world through its wisdom* did not come to know God, God was well-pleased through the foolishness of the message preached to save those who believe. For indeed Jews ask for signs, and Greeks search for *wisdom*; but we preach Christ crucified, to Jews a stumbling block, and to Gentiles foolishness, but to those who are the called, both Jews and Greeks, Christ the power of God and the *wisdom* of God. Because the foolishness of God is *wiser* than men, and the weakness of God is stronger than men. For consider your calling, brethren, that there were not many *wise* according to the flesh, not many mighty, not many noble; but God has chosen the foolish things of the world to shame the *wise*, and God has chosen the weak things of the world to shame the things which are strong (1:18-27; emphasis mine).

Again, in the next chapter, Paul goes on to say that when he preached to the Corinthians it was not with "superiority of speech or of *wisdom*" (1 Cor. 2:1), but rather "in demonstration of the Spirit and of power" (1 Cor. 2:4). These references to the wisdom of men as over against the wisdom of God are found all through chapter 2 (cf. vv. 5, 6, 7, 8, 13).

Much of the same may be said about "knowledge." Later in the book Paul writes:

Now concerning things sacrificed to idols, we know that we all have *knowledge*. *Knowledge* makes arrogant, but love edifies. If anyone supposes that he *knows* anything, he has not yet *known* as he ought to *know*; but if anyone loves God, he is *known* by Him (1 Cor. 8:1-3; emphasis mine).

Additional references to "knowledge" are found in verses 4, 7, 10, and 11 (see also 13:2, 8). Again we see how the knowledge of the world, as exemplified in Corinth, is arrogant and prideful and is an obstacle to the true knowledge of God.

What I am driving at is that when Paul comes to chapter 12, he "rescues both terms [wisdom and knowledge] from the Corinthian pneumatics and gives them a fresh stamp."[15] This leads me to believe that when it comes to defining these two spiritual gifts, we should do so in a manner consistent with Paul's argument in earlier portions of the epistle. I believe Dunn is correct to suggest that by "word of wisdom" Paul probably means "some charismatic utterance giving an insight into, some fresh understanding of God's plan of salvation or of the benefits it brings to believers."[16] Likewise, I agree with Gordon Fee who defines the "word of knowledge" as "something more akin to inspired teaching, perhaps related to receiving Christian insight into the meaning of Scripture."[17] I am not ruling out that God might communicate to someone information concerning the cause and nature of an illness. But it is highly unlikely that Paul has that in view when he talks about a word of wisdom and a word of knowledge. The wisdom and knowledge God imparts to his church through these spiritual gifts is in direct opposition to the spurious wisdom and knowledge of the world. The world thinks it is wise and knowledgeable in the things pertaining to man and the cosmos. But true wisdom and true knowledge come only from God as he illumines our minds to understand and appreciate the marvelous work he has done for us in Christ. This, I believe, is the nature and purpose of these two spiritual gifts.

Gifts of Healings (1 Cor. 12:9, 28)

Little needs to be said about gifts of healing, for Paul is simply describing that provision of spiritual power by which certain individuals in the body of Christ were enabled to effect physical wholeness in others. We saw this in operation on several occasions in the book of Acts, particularly through Peter and Paul.

The fact that both "gifts" and "healings" are plural has prompted some discussion. Some have seen that as Paul's way of telling us that there was no single power of healing effective for all illnesses. Rather there were many different gifts or powers of healing, each appropriate to and effective for its related illness. In other words, unlike Jesus, no single person in the church was endowed with a power or gift for healing every kind of disease. Richard Sipley offers a slightly different interpretation. "Each sign healing is a separate and individual gift given by God. The healing *itself* is the gift! Therefore through a certain Christian, God sovereignly produces different kinds of healing according to His own wisdom and will."[18]

Epaphroditus (Phil. 2:25-30)

A remarkable man of God, Epaphroditus was evidently sent by the church at Philippi to the apostle Paul bearing a substantial financial gift (cf. 4:18). Upon fulfilling his commission, he stayed with Paul to minister to him in whatever way proved necessary.

While serving at Paul's side, Epaphroditus apparently became ill, almost died, and was later healed by God. He is now being sent back to Philippi as the bearer of this epistle.

Note carefully what Paul says about him. Rarely, if ever, has the apostle spoken so highly of another man. "But I thought it necessary to send to you Epaphroditus," says Paul, "my brother and fellow-worker and fellow-soldier, who is also your messenger and minister to my need" (v. 25). If work needed to be done, Epaphroditus did it. If a spiritual battle needed to be fought, Epaphroditus fought it. If Paul was in any need, Epaphroditus met it.

But his love and concern did not stop with Paul. The apostle says that "he was longing for you all and was distressed because you [Philippians] had heard that he was sick" (v. 26). Did you read that correctly? Such was the depth and fervor of his love for them that Epaphroditus was worried lest the Philippians worry about him! Most of us fall into self-pity when we are sick, and we are probably a little resentful if others do not show us the care and concern we think we deserve. But not Epaphroditus. He is utterly selfless in his affliction, thinking only of the burden and heartache it might cause his brothers in Christ back in Philippi!

Paul says that Epaphroditus's warm-hearted love for the Philippians almost made him lose his mind! According to verse 26, he was "distressed," a word that implies a strong, deep, and disturbing upheaval in one's spirit. Far from feeling gratified that he was the object of so much concern back home, Epaphroditus was driven to mental torment with the thought that he might be a source of grief to his Christian brethren!

Paul's praise for Epaphroditus continues. He instructs the Philippians to receive him back with all joy and to "hold men like him in high regard, because he came close to death for the work of Christ, risking his life to complete what was deficient in your service to me" (vv. 29-30). The word Paul uses here that is translated "risking" is both rare and important. Gerald Hawthorne says that "from this word alone it is clear that Epaphroditus was no coward, but a courageous person willing to take enormous risks, ready to play with very high stakes in order to come to the aid of a person in need. He did not 'save' his life, but rather hazarded it to do for Paul and the cause of Christ what other Philippian Christians did not or could not do."[19] This is the kind of man, says the apostle, whom we should honor. He is the epitome of the selfless, loving, sacrificial servant of Jesus Christ.

Now you may be wondering why I have gone to such great lengths to emphasize the godly character of this man. The reason is simple enough. Charismatics must somehow account for why Epaphroditus became sick. Richard Sipley and Hugh Jeter, for example, suggest that Epaphroditus was sick because he sinned by overworking and consequently abusing his body.[20] But if that were so, it would have been ludicrous for Paul to have praised him as he did. Rather than speculate about what Paul did *not* say concerning Epaphroditus, we should build our case on what he *did* say. Paul is explicit with regard to both the motive and the ministry of this man of God. His behavior was beyond reproach. If he had fallen sick because of his own sin, would Paul have held him up as a model of Christian godliness? Would that all God's people might work as hard and as self-sacrificially as did this man from Philippi!

So why did Epaphroditus get sick? Why was he, in Paul's words, "a near neighbor to death" (v. 30)? We don't know. We *do* know that it was *not* because of sin or some flaw of faith. We can only surmise that God's purpose for Epaphroditus, Paul, and the Philippians, whatever that purpose might have been, could best be accomplished only through the bodily affliction of this choice saint.

Several other questions are appropriate. When Epaphroditus first became ill, why did not Paul heal him? Could not Paul simply have claimed his healing as a right due unto one for whom Jesus had died? If *anyone* should have been spared suffering and immediately healed, it was Epaphroditus. Yet we know that he was ill for a considerable period of time. How do we know this? Very simply from the fact that the Philippians had heard of his illness and *he* had heard that *they* had heard (v. 26). If Paul wrote this letter from Rome, as most believe he did, considerable time would have elapsed while word of Epaphroditus's illness was taken back to Philippi, not to mention the time it took for a messenger to return to Rome with news of how the Philippians had responded to their brother's illness. As the crow flies, Rome was over six hundred miles from

Philippi. Several weeks, perhaps months, would have passed from the time Epaphroditus fell sick to the time he received word that the Philippians were grieving over his condition.

But why did he suffer so severely and for so long a time? Why didn't Paul heal him, as he had healed many others throughout his ministry (cf. Acts)? And if Paul could not heal him, why didn't he request that someone with the gift of healing in the church at Rome do so? We are delighted, of course, as was Paul (v. 27), that God eventually did heal him. But not immediately. The example of Epaphroditus seems clearly to dispel the charismatic assumptions that God always wills to heal and that sin is the cause of all sickness.

Trophimus (2 Tim. 4:20)

In the midst of his greetings to young Timothy, Paul mentions the fact that he left Trophimus "sick at Miletus" (2 Tim. 4:20). We know little else about this man, except that he is mentioned in Acts 20:4 as being among those who accompanied Paul to Macedonia, and again in Acts 21:29 as being with the apostle in Jerusalem.

We have no way of knowing why he was sick, or for how long, or whether he was healed, and if so, by whom or in what manner. Perhaps he was ill in spite of his godliness, as was Epaphroditus. Or he may have been ill because of some sin. We simply do not know and would be wise not to speculate. One wonders, nevertheless, why the apostle Paul left him in that condition. If the problem with Trophimus was traceable to some sin in his life, one would have expected Paul to deal with it. If it was not sin, one might have expected him to have healed his fellow-worker, or at least to have put him in contact with someone who could. Again we are left with the question, if God always wills to heal and if the gift of healing was still in operation, why was Trophimus "left sick at Miletus"?

Timothy (1 Tim. 5:23)

We have come to the famous passage in which Paul instructs Timothy, "No longer drink water exclusively, but use a little wine for the sake of your stomach and your frequent ailments."

Evidently Timothy practiced total abstinence, perhaps in defer-
ence to those who sought to bring some accusation against him.
While Paul tells him to keep himself "free from sin" (v. 22), he did
not mean that Timothy was to swear off the use of wine altogether.
But why did Paul recommend wine? J. N. D. Kelly tells us.

> The beneficial effects of wine as a remedy against dyspeptic
> complaints, as a tonic, and as counteracting the effects of im-
> pure water, were widely recognized in antiquity, and modern
> travellers in Mediterranean countries have confirmed its
> value for the third at any rate of these purposes. The author of
> Proverbs (xxxi. 6) advises its use for maladies of both body and
> soul; Hippocrates recommends moderate draughts of wine for
> a patient for whose stomach water alone is dangerous; and
> Plutarch states that wine is the most useful of drinks and the
> pleasantest of medicines.[21]

But if Timothy had stomach problems, why didn't Paul exercise
the gift of healing and put an end to it? Or again, if he could not,
surely someone Paul knew could have.

A more important question is why Timothy had stomach problems in the first place! And not only stomach problems, but "frequent ailments" according to Paul (v. 23). If Timothy's stomach
problems and frequent ailments were the results of recurrent sin,
why didn't Paul rebuke this young man and set him straight? If he
was such a repeat offender that he was *frequently* ailing, why did
Paul select him as his apostolic legate and representative? Surely
Paul could have chosen someone more spiritually qualified. If his
ailments were the result of a lack of faith or a failure to pray, why
didn't Paul call him to repentance? However, if his illnesses were
not due to sin, why didn't Paul instruct him to do what modern
charismatics recommend: claim his healing and disregard his
symptoms? Instead, Paul commends Timothy's performance and
character repeatedly throughout both epistles addressed to him.
There is every indication that Paul looked upon Timothy's physical maladies, as well as his own, as par for the course. He advises
his young friend, as he would undoubtedly advise us, to take ad-
vantage of every legitimate medicinal remedy to alleviate discom-

fort. Paul was neither shocked nor dismayed by Timothy's ailment. Neither should we be by ours.

3 John 2

"Beloved," writes John the apostle to his friend Gaius, "I pray that in all respects you may prosper and be in good health, just as your soul prospers." Earlier, in chapter 2, I commented that Hebrews 13:8 and Isaiah 53:4-5 are perhaps the two most important passages for the healing movement today. This passage in John's third epistle isn't far behind. Hugh Jeter is typical of most charismatics when he says, on the basis of this verse, that "God wants His children to be physically healthy. He wants us to 'prosper and be in health' (3 John 2), as long as our souls also prosper."[22]

This faulty interpretation could have been avoided if careful consideration had been given to the nature of New Testament epistles. For what we have in this verse is simply a standard form of greeting found in most letters of the ancient world.[23] Gordon Fee reminds us that "just as there is a standard form to our letters (date, salutation, body, close, and signature), so there was for theirs [i.e., the ancients]. Thousands of ancient letters have been found, and most of them have a form exactly like those in the New Testament."[24] One of the standard elements in such letters is the health-wish, such as we find here in 3 John 2. To argue that this typical salutation provides a basis for a theology of health and wealth for all Christians in every age would be ridiculous.

That of course, does not mean that praying and hoping for the good health and financial prosperity of our fellow believers is wrong. In this passage John prays that Gaius might "prosper," a verb that literally means "to be led along a good road" or "to have a good journey." Here it is used metaphorically to "prosper," or "succeed" (cf. Rom. 1:10; 1 Cor. 16:2). But to say that was John's wish for Gaius is not at all to demonstrate that it is always God's will for everyone.

John also desires that Gaius be in good health. We cannot know for certain whether this means that Gaius was suffering from bad health. Remember, this was a standard greeting. As I. Howard

Marshall has said, "The phrase would be perfectly possible in a letter to somebody with robust health, that he may continue to enjoy it."[25] But if Gaius was indeed ill, that would merely confirm what we have found in other biblical passages—that a believer who is prospering spiritually can at the same time be suffering physically. For John's prayer is that Gaius would prosper physically "just as" (or "even as") his soul is prospering. There can be no doubt that Gaius was a godly man, as verses 3-8 make clear. John's desire for his friend is that his body would make as much progress as his soul. And that should be our prayer for our brethren as well. Whether or not it is God's desire is something we cannot know.

11

PAUL'S THORN IN THE FLESH

Paul's thorn in the flesh, whatever it was, has proved to be an especially bothersome thorn in the side of the modern healing movement. On the surface it seems to run counter to several crucial doctrines they espouse. If sickness is never the will of God for the saints, if God is never glorified by their perseverance in pain, how does one account for the experience of the apostle Paul? Most charismatics do not believe that Paul's "thorn" was a physical illness. They offer another explanation, which I'll explain shortly. But a few in the healing movement concede that Paul suffered from an unrelenting physical malady. They insist, however, that his experience was an exception to the general rule that God wants us wholly healthy.

What does the Bible say about Paul's "thorn in the flesh," and what does his experience tell us about our own?

The Purpose of Paul's "Thorn"

To make sense of Paul's suffering we must first consider the context in which it appears. The larger context of Paul's comments is, of course, the book of 2 Corinthians as a whole. In this epistle, more so than in any other, Paul is compelled against his will to defend his apostolic authority. He finds it a distasteful and foolish task (cf. 10:8, 17-18; 11:1, 16-21, 30; 12:5-6), but the well-being of the Christians in Corinth is at stake. They have left him no choice. "Boasting is necessary," says Paul, "though it is not profitable" (12:1). If those who question his authority are demanding apostolic credentials, he will provide them, not least of which are the "visions and revelations of the Lord" granted him (12:1).

Paul describes in 2 Corinthians 12:1-6 what may well have been the most remarkable experience of his apostolic career. He tells of an occasion when he was mysteriously and suddenly translated into Paradise, where he "heard inexpressible words, which a man is not permitted to speak" (12:4). Nowhere do we read of this sort of thing happening to anyone other than Paul. (The closest parallel would be the experience of John in the book of Revelation.) Thus it was perfectly suited to generate pride in his apostolic, though still sinful, heart. But the Lord would not stand for it and therefore gave Paul "a bridle that held him back from haughtiness."[1] Paul put it this way: "And because of the surpassing greatness of the revelations, for this reason, to keep me from exalting myself, there was given me a thorn in the flesh, a messenger of Satan to buffet me — to keep me from exalting myself!" (12:7).

The Source of Paul's "Thorn"

Where did Paul's thorn in the flesh come from? Or perhaps we should ask, From *whom* did it come? The subject of the verb is left unexpressed ("there was given me"), a fact that some charismatic authors have tried to use to deny that God had anything to do with this affair. But virtually every commentator I have consulted agrees that this is another example of what is called "the divine passive," in which God is "the hidden agent behind events and experiences in human lives."[2] In other words, we have here "a conventional use of the passive voice to avoid mentioning the divine name."[3] Had Paul wanted to say that Satan was the source, he probably would not have used the Greek verb *didōmi*. As Ralph Martin points out, "This word was usually employed to denote that God's favor had been bestowed (cf. Gal. 3:21; Eph. 3:8; 5:19; 1 Tim. 4:14)."[4] If Satan were the ultimate source of the thorn, other, more appropriate Greek verbs were available to express that thought.[5]

There are several other important points in this passage. For example, the word translated "thorn" is found only here in all of the New Testament. In classical Greek it was used with reference to a pointed stake on which the head of an enemy was impaled after decapitation. More commonly, though, it simply referred to a splinter or thorn stuck in the body. Paul apparently envisions himself impaled by this affliction, pinned, as it were, to the ground and thus rendered helpless by it. This must have been an excruciating malady, for "an apostle who could willingly put up with the sufferings and deprivations listed in 2 Corinthians 11 would not beseech the Lord so strenuously and repeatedly for the removal of some minor problem that could easily be borne."[6]

This thorn is further described as a "messenger [literally, an "angel"] of Satan." Elsewhere in Scripture we see instances in which God employs the devil to accomplish his will (cf. Job; 1 Cor. 5:5). Not everyone, however, is willing to concede this point. God and Satan, so we are told, always work at cross purposes. If Satan wants it, God doesn't, and vice versa. That is ultimately true, of course. But we must remember that God and Satan can both desire the same event to occur, while hoping to accomplish through it antithetical results. Satan certainly wanted to see Jesus crucified, as did God the Father (Isa. 53:10; Acts 2:23; 4:27-28). But they obviously wanted it for different reasons. The situation with Job is another case in point. Satan afflicted him only by divine permission. What Satan had hoped would destroy Job (or at least provoke him to blasphemy), God used to strengthen him.

We have much the same thing here. We do not know if this messenger of Satan was acting consciously in the service of God or with his express permission, as in the case of Job. More than likely we are to understand that by God's secret and sovereign providence a demonic being was dispatched to Paul intent on oppressing and thereby hindering (or even destroying) his ministry. The divine design, however, was to keep Paul from sinful pride and to utilize this affliction to accomplish a higher spiritual good (cf. 12:9-10). God often does use Satan to accomplish his goals, sometimes with and sometimes without Satan's knowledge of it. Joni Eareckson Tada explains it beautifully and makes application of this truth to her own experience.

> Satan intends the rain which ruins a church picnic to cause the people to curse their Lord; but God uses the rain to develop their patience. Satan plans to hinder the work of an

effective missionary by arranging for him to trip and break a leg; God allows the accident so that the missionary's patient response to the pain and discomfort will bring glory to Himself. Satan brews a hurricane to kill thousands in a small Indian village so he can enjoy the misery and destruction; God uses the storm to display His awesome power, to show people the awful consequences that sin has brought to the world, to drive some to search for Him, to harden others in their sin, and to remind us that He is free to do as He pleases—that we will never figure Him out. Satan schemed that a seventeen-year-old girl named Joni would break her neck, hoping to ruin her life; God sent the broken neck in answer to her prayer for a closer walk with Him and uses her wheelchair as a platform to display His sustaining grace.[7]

Remember that the purpose of Paul's affliction was "to buffet me—to keep me from exalting myself" (12:7).[8] There may well be some significance in Paul's use of the present tense of the verb "to buffet" (literally, "to beat or strike a blow with the fist"; cf. Matt. 26:67). It may be his way of telling us that the affliction recurred periodically throughout his life and was even at this time bearing down heavily and painfully on him. This is confirmed in verse 8 where Paul says he prayed three times that he might be delivered. Perhaps the affliction had flared up on three distinct occasions when its humiliating effect would have been most evident. Then again, the reference to his threefold prayer may simply be Paul's way of comparing his own nonredemptive suffering to that of the Lord Jesus in Gethsemane.

The Nature of Paul's "Thorn"

What was this "thorn in the flesh"? Many, if not most, charismatics in our day argue for an interpretation first defended by Chrysostom in the fourth century. On this view, Paul's "thorn" is simply a reference to all the enemies of the Christian gospel who opposed and persecuted him during his evangelistic and theological labors. The names of Alexander the coppersmith (2 Tim. 4:14) and Hymenaeus and Philetus (2 Tim. 2:17) are the first to come to mind. "Thorn in the flesh," therefore, is a collective and obviously figurative expression for all of Paul's adversaries. Writes R. V. G. Tasker:

> As there is nothing which tends to elate a Christian evan-
> gelist so much as the enjoyment of spiritual experiences, and
> as there is nothing so calculated to deflate the spiritual pride
> which may follow them as the opposition he encounters while
> preaching the word, it is not unlikely that Chrysostom's inter-
> pretation is nearer the truth than any other.[9]

Those who argue for this position appeal to 2 Corinthians 11:14-15 where Paul's opponents are described as the "servants" (literally, "ministers") of Satan, who is himself "an angel of light." They are also quick to remind us that in the Greek translation of the Old Testament (the Septuagint, or LXX) this word translated "thorn" is twice used metaphorically of one's enemies (Num. 33:55; Ezek. 28:24). Therefore, when Paul says "thorn in the flesh," he means something similar to our modern idiom "a pain in the neck."

Whereas the Greek word for "thorn" may, in the LXX, be used metaphorically of one's enemies, the question is whether that is its use in 2 Corinthians 12. The evidence strongly indicates otherwise.

First, the singular "a messenger of Satan" is hardly a clear and unmistakable way to refer to an entire group of persons. If Paul had in mind a group of opponents, he chose an especially obscure way to make his point.

Second, Paul has already made it clear in 2 Corinthians 4:7-15; 6:9-10; and particularly in 11:23-28 that opposition and persecution are normal for *every* person in gospel ministry. No servant of Christ is exempt from either Satanic or human resistance. The an-tagonism Paul encountered when he preached the gospel is an ex-perience common to all Christian believers. Yet Paul describes his "thorn" as something uniquely his, given to him for a particular reason subsequent to a truly singular event (cf. 12:1-6).

The third reason I find the charismatic view inadequate pertains to chronology. Paul says that the thorn was given him sometime after his translation into Paradise, an event he explicitly dates as having occurred "fourteen years ago" (12:2). Since we know that 2 Corinthians was written in either late A.D. 55 or early 56, Paul could have received his thorn no earlier than A.D. 41-42, a full eight years after his conversion to Christ.[10] Yet we know from Acts 9:23-30 and elsewhere that Paul encountered Satanically inspired opposition to his ministry from the very moment of his conversion.

Fourth, Paul's prayer in verse 8 militates against this interpretation. "Would the apostle pray to be spared persecution? This is doubtful, since persecution was the fuel on which Paul seemed to thrive. The more he was persecuted, the more he seemed determined to press the claims of his apostolate."[11] And let us never forget that Paul knew better than anyone (cf. 2 Cor. 2:12-17) that the success of the gospel he proclaimed was not in his power to control. It, like everything in his life and ministry, was under the providential oversight of God. In view of these facts, it is unlikely that Paul had in mind his opponents, when he spoke of his thorn in the flesh.

A popular view among Roman Catholic interpreters during the Middle Ages was that Paul's "thorn" referred to inordinate sexual desire, i.e., *lust*. But would God have told Paul to cease praying for deliverance from sexual lust? Would Paul himself have boasted about sexual weakness (cf. 12:9), or acquiesced contentedly to its power in his life (cf. 12:10)? Certainly not! Furthermore, this view conflicts with Paul's declaration in 1 Corinthians 7:1-9 that he had been gifted with the strength of celibacy.

John Calvin suggested that the word "thorn" was designed "to sum up all the different kinds of trials with which Paul was exercised."[12] C. K. Barrett thinks it was a speech impediment, perhaps a stutter. Others have suggested epilepsy, malaria, gallstones, kidney stones, gout, deafness, dental infection, rheumatism, earaches, headaches, sciatica, arthritis, and even leprosy!

If his thorn was indeed a physical malady, as I believe it was, the most cogent explanation is that he suffered from a severe case of ophthalmia or conjunctivitis. In Galatians 4:13-15 Paul said, "But you [Galatian Christians] know that it was because of a bodily illness that I preached the gospel to you the first time; and that which was a trial to you in my bodily condition you did not despise or loathe, but you received me as an angel of God, as Christ Jesus Himself. Where then is that sense of blessing you had? For I bear you witness, that if possible, you would have plucked out your eyes and given them to me." Evidently Paul suffered from a painful bodily affliction that was especially humiliating, because loathsome and repulsive to others. Although the statement in verse 15 may only be figurative, emphasizing the sacrificial love the Galatians had for Paul, it is just as likely an indication that this loathsome illness from which he suffered was related to his eyes.

Lessons Paul Learned

Although the exact nature of Paul's affliction remains shrouded in ambiguity, its purpose is perfectly clear. The thorn was given him, says J. I. Packer, "not for punishment, but for protection. Physical weakness guarded him against spiritual sickness."[13] Bodily pain, says Charles Hodge, has different effects on different people:

> In the unrenewed its tendency is to exasperate; when self-inflicted its tendency is to debase and fill the soul with grovelling ideas of God and religion, and with low self-conceit. But when inflicted by God on his own children, it more than any thing teaches them to submit when submission is most difficult. Though he slay me, [yet] I will trust in him, is the expression of the highest form of faith.[14]

In brief, the more we hurt, the more we lean. Paul certainly learned this lesson well.

He learned other lessons also, lessons that each of us ought to consider. His ailment taught him something about divine providence and how to respond to it. Paul's reaction in verse 9, once the Lord had declined his request three times over, was not one of stoical resignation to an inexorable fate. His response was not a sullen "Que sera, sera," but a joyful delight in the privilege of being an instrument for the manifestation of Christ's power.

Paul was also taught the proper perspective on human suffering and weakness. One is to be "well content with weaknesses, with insults, with distresses, with persecutions, with difficulties, for Christ's sake" (12:10), for "the greater the servant's weakness, the more conspicuous is the power of His Master's all-sufficient grace."[15] This does not mean that we are to seek out suffering on our own.

Paul is not encouraging some morbid self-imposed asceticism. His afflictions were *God-given* for *Christ's* sake. Paul's joy was not in pain, but in his realization of the complete adequacy of God's grace in Christ both to meet his every need and to transform his weaknesses into a stage on which the glory and power of Christ might be displayed. R. V. G. Tasker puts it well:

> Only a morbid fanatic can take pleasure in the sufferings he inflicts upon himself; only an insensitive fool can take pleasure in the sufferings that are the consequences of his folly; and only a convinced Christian can take pleasure in sufferings endured *for Christ's sake*, for he alone has been initiated into the divine secret, that it is only when he is *weak*, having thrown himself unreservedly in penitence and humility upon the never-failing mercies of God, that he is *strong*, with a strength not his own, but belonging to the "Lord of all power and might."[16]

Paul also learned that the Christian life is not designed as an opportunity for us to experience and display our own power and prestige. It is designed to magnify the power of God, which may well demand that we endure severe weakness. To come right to the point, God doesn't exist for us; we exist for him.

Finally, Paul also learned that his purity is more important than pleasure. Of greater value to God than Paul's happiness was Paul's holiness. If, in the divine wisdom, it was necessary to give him pain in order to protect him from pride, Paul was willing to yield to the divine purpose. If, as God saw things, the best way to make Paul humble was to make him hurt, so be it. That was the spirit of the apostle. May it be ours as well.

12

ANOINTING WITH OIL
AND THE PRAYER OF FAITH

The news from the Persian Gulf was not very encouraging on the day I began working on this chapter. The Iranians stood poised to attack. The Iraqis were prepared to retaliate. The United States had dispatched battleships and sophisticated mine-sweeping devices to protect Kuwaiti tankers as they cautiously made their way through the strait of Ormuz. You may wonder, Why? What is so important about the Persian Gulf? What could possibly explain why so many would risk so much, perhaps even war? The answer, in one word, is *oil*. The songwriter was mistaken. It isn't *love* that makes the world go 'round, it's *oil*! Many people dig for it, some even die for it. Others spend vast sums of money to guarantee that our supply of it continues unabated. Such is the age in which we live.

Oil was obviously important in the Middle East two thousand years ago, although I seriously doubt that anyone would have died for it! It was oil of a different kind, certainly not the "black gold" of which dreams are made and empires built. James, the half-brother of Jesus, had some interesting comments about the use of oil in the early church. If anyone fell sick, wrote James, he should summon the elders of the church who would not only pray for him but also anoint him with oil in the name of the Lord (James 5:14). Having done so, James assured his readers that "the prayer offered in faith will restore the one who is sick, and the Lord will raise him up, and if he has committed sins, they will be forgiven him" (James 5:15).

Anointing With Oil

Our concern obviously is not with the financial and political power of Texas crude, but with the religious significance of what was probably common olive oil. Why did James give instructions that the sick were to be anointed with oil? What effect, if any, did it have on their healing? Should we literally follow James's instructions today? These are a few of the questions that need to be answered as we turn our attention to this important and controversial passage.

Not everyone believes that James was talking about physical illness. For example, Daniel R. Hayden suggests that James was addressing the problem of "emotional distress and spiritual exhaustion experienced by God's people in their deep struggle with temptation and their relentless battle with besetting sin."[1] He points out that the Greek word translated "sick" in verse 14 (astheneō) can mean "weak" in faith or spiritually fatigued (cf. Rom. 14:1, 2; 1 Cor. 8:11, 12; 2 Cor. 13:3), as is also true of the other Greek word translated "sick" in verse 15 (kamnō; cf. Heb. 12:3). It is also true that the Greek words in verses 15-16 translated "restore" (sōzō), "raise up" (egeirō), and "heal" (iaomai) may legitimately refer to the restoration or renewal of spiritual and emotional vitality. These observations indicate that the view under consideration is at least possible.

But is that probable? Douglas Moo thinks not, and reminds us that "while astheneō can denote spiritual weakness, this meaning is usually made clear by a qualifier (cf. Rom. 14:2, 'in faith'; 1 Cor. 8:7, 'in conscience') or the context. Moreover, in the material that is most relevant to James, the Gospels, astheneō almost always refers to illness. The same is true for kamnō. And iaomai, when not used in an Old Testament quotation, always refers in the New Testament to physical healing."[2] As far as sōzō and egeirō are concerned, both are appropriate descriptions of physical healing (sōzō in Matt. 9:21-22; Mark 5:34; 6:56; 10:52; Luke 7:50; 17:19; and egeirō in Mark 1:31; 2:9-12; Acts 3:7). Therefore, while we certainly should not ignore this interpretation, I am going to proceed on the assumption that James has in mind physical illness.

I find it interesting that James does not tell the sick person to pray for healing (although I am sure it would have been okay). Rather, he encourages him to call the elders of the church in order that *they* might pray over him. James does not tell him to call for someone with the spiritual gift of healing. Nor does he recommend that he attend a healing service or be brought publicly before the church. But why are the elders of the church singled out? It isn't because they alone were thought to have the gift of healing. Nowhere in the New Testament lists of qualifications for elders is the gift of healing mentioned as a requirement for office (cf. Titus 1 and 1 Tim. 3). Perhaps they are mentioned because they functioned not only as leaders but also as representatives of the entire body of Christ in its ministry to the hurting and lost. It may also be because the elders of the church were generally men of deep spiritual experience and maturity. They especially should be able to pray "in faith." (Note that the prayer in response to which God heals the man is that of the *elders*, not the sick person.) Whatever the reason, one should not conclude that *only* elders are responsible to pray for the sick. In verse 16 James tells the entire church, "Confess your sins to one another, and pray for one another, so that you may be healed."

As the elders pray for the sick, they are to anoint him with oil in the name of the Lord. Aside from Mark 6:13 this is the only passage in the New Testament that recommends the use of oil for the sick. In other words, the great majority of healings described in the New Testament were accomplished *without* oil. That would suggest that while it is certainly permissible to anoint the sick with oil when we pray for them, it is not absolutely necessary.

But why did James mention the use of oil at all? Some believe he was recommending it as a medicinal aid. You may recall that when the Good Samaritan ministered to the man who had been beaten and robbed, he "came to him, and bandaged up his wounds, pouring oil and wine on them" (Luke 10:34). It is common knowledge that oil was frequently used in the ancient world for medicinal purposes. This may account for James's use of the verb *aleiphō* ("to anoint"), which emphasizes the actual physical action of pouring. Another word that means "to anoint" (*chriō*) is usually employed when the purpose of the anointing is religious or symbolic. However, the distinction between these two verbs for anointing should not be pressed, for their meanings often overlap.[3] But if the oil in James 5 was strictly medicinal, why is it *alone* mentioned as a helpful remedy for the sick? Oil was no doubt beneficial, but no one claims it was appropriate for *every* illness. Also, if the purpose of the oil was exclusively medicinal, why was it necessary for the elders to do the anointing? Would not others, or perhaps the individual himself, have already done this to alleviate his suffering?

Perhaps then the oil has a religious significance in this passage. In that case it would probably symbolize the Holy Spirit and his ministry of consecration whereby an individual or some object is set aside to God's service (cf. 1 Sam. 16:13; Isa. 61:1; Acts 4:27). I am inclined to agree with Moo who views the anointing "as a physical action with symbolic significance. Since the symbolism of 'anointing' is usually associated with the setting apart or consecrating of someone or something to God, we are probably to understand this as the symbolism intended in the action. As the elders pray for the sick person, they also set that person apart for God's special attention."[4]

The important thing to remember is that it is not the oil or any spiritual power it might contain that accounts for the man's restoration to health. James is very clear on this point. He says it is the *prayer* offered in faith that restores the sick and that *God* will raise him up. But what is "the prayer of faith"?

The Prayer of Faith

In his commentary on James, D. Edmond Hiebert insists that "the prayer offered in faith" is not just any prayer that may be prayed any time, but a unique and divinely motivated one. He appeals to the definite article ("the") before both "prayer" and "faith," giving us the translation, "*the* prayer of *the* faith." His contention is that God enables a man (or the elders) to pray this prayer only in special circumstances. It therefore "is not just an ordinary prayer for another, however good and sincere it may be, but the prayer prompted by the Spirit-wrought conviction that it is the Lord's will to heal the one being prayed for."[5]

That is much like the view of Douglas Moo, although Moo does not base any of his argument on the definite article ("the"). A prayer uttered in faith, says Moo, "always includes within it a tacit acknowledgment of God's sovereignty in all matters; that it is *God's* will that must be done. And it is clear that it is by no means always God's will to heal those who are ill (cf. 2 Cor. 12:7-9). There-fore, the 'faith' that is the indispensable condition for our prayers for healing to be answered — this faith being the gift of God — can be truly present only when it is God's will to heal."[6] In others words:

> The faith with which we pray is always faith in the God whose will is supreme and best; only sometimes does this faith include assurance that a particular request is within that will. . . . Prayer for healing offered in the confidence that God will answer that prayer *does* bring healing; but only when it is God's will to heal will that faith, itself a gift of God, be pres-ent. Such faith cannot be "manufactured," however gifted, in-sistent, or righteous we are. In this life, we shall not, most of the time, be able to know whether God's will is to heal; we shall not always be able to sense whether that "faith" that gets what is asked for is present. When our sincere, fervent prayers for healing go unanswered, therefore, it is not our lack of faith that is at fault; the context in which such faith could be pres-ent was absent.[7]

The key, then, is remembering that faith is first and fundamen-tally a divine gift. It is a work of grace, not a product of our own efforts, be they ever so earnest. It may just be that the Lord wishes to suspend certain blessings on the condition of faith, a faith that *he alone* can supply. That anyone should ever exercise this kind of faith can only be because God has produced it in his heart. When God wishes to heal a person on the condition of wholehearted belief, he himself produces that belief in the heart of the one who prays. Therefore, the particular kind of faith to which James is re-ferring, in response to which God will grant our request, is not the kind that we may exercise at *our* will. It is the kind of faith that we exercise only when *God* wills.

James makes one additional comment of immense significance. He says, "And if he [the sick man] has committed sins, they will be forgiven him" (James 5:15). James obviously agrees with Jesus (John 9:1-3) and Paul (2 Cor. 12:1-10) that not all sickness is the direct result of sin. Sometimes it is (cf. 1 Cor. 11:27-30; and perhaps Mark 2:1-12), but not always. The "if" in verse 15 is not designed to say this man may *never* have sinned. "The meaning seems to be that, if God should effect a miraculous cure in answer to the elders' prayer of faith accompanied by anointing with oil in the name of the Lord, that would be a clear indication that any sins of the sufferer, which might have been responsible for this particular illness, were forgiven."[8] In other words, *if* sin was responsible for his sickness, the fact that God heals him physically is evidence that God has forgiven him spiritually.

We have learned from James 5 that prayer for the sick is of crucial importance, not only in the ministry of the elders of the church but also on the part of the congregation as a whole. We also have seen that oil *may* be used as a symbol of the work of the Holy Spirit in consecrating the afflicted person for God's special care, but that in *most* descriptions of healing in the New Testament it is absent. This passage also teaches us that when God wills to heal someone, he may sometimes inspire and cultivate in those who are praying the unassailable assurance ("faith") that such is indeed his will. Finally, James makes it clear that illness *may* be the result of sin, but need not be. If it is, God's healing of the person is a visible sign of his forgiveness as well.

Should we today pray for the sick? Absolutely! Should we today anoint the sick with oil? It is certainly permissible, if they so desire. Will God today heal those for whom we pray? Yes, if it is his will to do so.

13

"WHY YOU LORD?" OR, SUFFERING AND GOD'S PROVIDENCE

My secretary just stuck her head in my office to tell me that an earthquake of major proportions (6.1 on the Richter scale) hit southern California at 7:45 A.M. Pacific time. There were four aftershocks, but as yet the full extent of the damage is unknown. My thoughts turned immediately to the countless individuals who would undoubtedly suffer greatly from that disaster.

Any time there is suffering like that, whether physical, financial, or emotional, we always ask the same questions: Where is God? Why does he permit this to happen? What am I going to do now? If he is behind it all, is he worthy of my worship? Often our immediate response is to quote Romans 8:28: "And we know that God causes all things to work together for good to those who love God, to those who are called according to His purpose." We get a lot of mileage out of that verse, sometimes pressing it into service like a divinely inspired pacifier. When people cry or complain about their suffering, we plug Romans 8:28 into their mouths to calm them down. But will it? What does this passage really tell us about suffering and God and our desperate need to be comforted and consoled?

My understanding of this marvelous verse of Scripture is that it functions less as a pacifier and more as a loving, concerned parent who takes a hurting child into his or her arms and tenderly cuddles him, whispering words of reassurance and affection. For that is how God deals with us in our pain. Let's look at Romans 8:28 word by word and see if we can come to an appreciation of why we suffer and what God is doing about it.

"We know"

The first thing that strikes me about this passage is Paul's confidence. He says we *know* that God causes all things to work together for good. There isn't the slightest doubt in his mind about God's role in our pain. There are no questions, no second guesses. He doesn't say "we *wish*" or "we *hope*," but "we *know*" that God causes all things to work together for good. How does Paul know? What is the source of his certainty? The answer is in verses 29-30. There he tells us that since God's loving purpose for our salvation stretches from eternity past into eternity future, there is nothing that can ultimately do us any spiritual harm. In other words, the reason we *know* that all things work together for our ultimate spiritual profit is that God loved us before the foundation of the world and predestined us to be conformed to the image of his Son! And those whom he predestined he called, and those whom he called, he justified, and those whom he justified he glorified! God has an eternal and personal stake in your spiritual welfare and will not permit anyone or anything to interfere with his plan for your life. You may rest assured that nothing comes your way, no matter how painful, no matter how persistent, that can ultimately do you any harm. God is determined to bring you safely into his heavenly kingdom and nothing can thwart his purpose.

"that"

The second thing you should note about this verse is what Paul does *not* say. He does not say, "And we know *how* God works all things together for good." There is a world of difference between knowing *that* God does something and knowing *how* he does it. When Paul uses the word "that" instead of "how," he is telling us that although our knowledge in this matter is certain, it is not exhaustive. We may speak with absolute confidence concerning God's providential power to bring good out of bad. But we will rarely be in a position to explain how he did it.

This poses a very real problem, for the simple fact that few people are willing to settle for that kind of knowledge. It isn't enough to tell them *that* God will use their pain for spiritual profit; they want to know *how* he intends to do so. They want to see for themselves precisely how and in what ways adversity and suffering and conflict and confusion work together for good. When tragedy hits us hard, we want to know right then and there, immediately, why it happened and what possible good can come from it. Of course, sometimes we can figure it out. But that is usually after the fact, with the benefit of hindsight. Rarely do we perceive the divine purpose before it happens.

If nothing else this fact ought to keep us from prying into those secrets of God's purpose which he has not chosen to reveal (cf. Deut. 29:29). John Calvin put it well:

> But we must so cherish moderation that we do not try to make God render account to us, but so reverence his secret judgments as to consider his will the truly just cause of all things. When dense clouds darken the sky, and a violent tempest arises, because a gloomy mist is cast over our eyes, thunder strikes our ears and all our senses are benumbed with fright, everything seems to us to be confused and mixed up; but all the while a constant quiet and serenity ever remain in heaven. So we must infer that, while the disturbances in the world deprive us of judgment [i.e., understanding], God out of the pure light of his justice and wisdom tempers and directs these very movements in the best-conceived order to a right end.[1]

In other words, some things that God does are none of our business! We need to be careful not to poke our theological noses into places they don't belong. Our faith in God and our obligation to serve him do not depend on our ability to figure out the mysteries of his providence. God is worthy of our trust and devotion regardless of what may befall us, regardless of how much or little we may understand about it.

"God"

Notice, third, that it is *God* who works all things together for good. I say this in spite of the omission of the word "God" in a number of ancient Greek manuscripts, which thus read "And we know that all things work together for good." But if "God" was not part of the original text, what reason do we have for proceeding as if it were?

There are several reasons. In the first place, Paul says in the latter part of the verse that we are called according to a *purpose*. But what is a "purpose"? A purpose is a conscious intent to accomplish a goal. In other words, a purpose implies a *purposer*, someone who *intends* to take the seemingly senseless things of life and make of them something profitable and lasting. Things in and of themselves do not think and formulate plans! Yet Paul says that all things work together for our good. How can that be unless it is God who providentially uses those things to accomplish his purpose? Furthermore, as we have already seen, the basis for Paul's confident assertion in verse 28 is the reality of the divine plan in verses 29-30. The reason we are assured that the things in this life work ultimately for our good is that God is working to bring us into conformity with his Son. And let us not forget that what Romans 8:28 says only implicitly, Ephesians 1:11 says explicitly. There Paul tells us that it is God "who works *all things* after the counsel of His will."

Paul's point is that our faith and confidence are in God, not in things. Have you ever caught yourself saying to someone who is suffering through difficult times, "Don't worry; I just know things will be all right." Or perhaps you have consoled them by saying, "Don't despair; these things just have a way of working themselves out in time." If you have, you need to go back and set matters straight with your friend. For, you see, "things" are subservient to God's providential will. If things do work out, if in time one's situation does improve, it is only because of God's marvelous, matchless control of every "thing" that exists.

"all things"

The "things" in our lives, both good and bad, are a lot like the pieces of a jigsaw puzzle. Try as we may, we are often unable to put all the pieces together. But God has the box top! He knows where every piece fits and in time will see that it is put there. Similarly life may seem like the underside of a tapestry, with no pattern, purpose, or resolution. We see only a confusing array of colors that make no apparent sense. But God sees things from the other side! From the vantage point of eternity he sees the beauty of that portrait, which is your life, because it is he who weaves every random thread into a meaningful whole.

But this all raises a crucial question about Romans 8:28. Just what are the "things" over which God exercises his control? Surely the context gives us at least a partial answer. In verse 17-18 Paul said that if we are children of God, then we are "heirs also, heirs of God and fellow-heirs with Christ, if indeed we suffer with Him in order that we may also be glorified with Him. For I consider that the sufferings of this present time are not worthy to be compared with the glory that is to be revealed to us." The "things" God causes to work together for good, therefore, are all the experiences that together constitute the suffering we endure for Christ's sake. Whatever form this suffering might take, whether bodily affliction, financial adversity, or emotional distress, we are to take comfort in knowing that God has it all under wraps.

In the context that follows Paul also mentions numerous things that in one way or another threaten, but fail, to sever us from the love of Christ. What are the "things" God causes to work together for our good? There is tribulation and distress and persecution and famine and nakedness and peril and sword, just to mention a few! As if that were not enough, there is death and life and angels and principalities and things present and things future, things above and things below. No created thing, anywhere of any kind, says Paul, can elude God's overruling providential power.

"work together"

There is still more to come! Paul says that we know God causes all things to *work together* for good. He does not say all things *are* good, but that God is more than capable of causing them to work together *for* good. Paul is not about to suggest that such things as disease and poverty and pain are good things. Nor does he say that

God *transforms* evil things into good things, in the sense that they cease to be evil once God has finished with them. What he says is that God can take something inherently evil and make it serve a higher, better, and more productive end. Although Joseph's brothers intended to bring him harm when they sold him into slavery in Egypt, "God meant it for good in order to bring about this present result, to preserve many people alive" (Gen. 50:20; cf. 45:1-8).

"for good"

A lot of people have been waiting anxiously for precisely this moment. They are eager to cash in on the "good" that Paul confidently promises will come from the things over which God exercises his control. They have it in their heads that "good" in Romans 8:28 is worldly comfort, possessions, power, or some such notion. But this verse does not mean that if we lose one job God will always give us a better one. It does not imply that if we become ill this week we will experience good health the next. The "good" that God brings out of the bad may not be recognizable as good, at least as we define the term. This verse is not a promise that God will bring riches out of poverty or laughter out of sorrow or pleasure out of pain.

I am persuaded that the "good" of Romans 8:28 is defined in Romans 8:29. There Paul says that God's design is to bring us into moral and spiritual conformity to the image of his Son, the Lord Jesus Christ! In other words, God's ultimate purpose in exercising providential control over the "all things" in our lives is to make us Christ-like. It is holiness, not health, and purity, not possessions, that God has promised.

"to those who love God"

Finally, we see that this promise is restricted. It is for "those who love God," for "those who are called according to His purpose." Surely God exercises sovereign control over the lives of both Christians and non-Christians. But no unbeliever can have assurance that any good will come from any "thing" he experiences. The promise, Paul says, is for those that love God.

That narrows the field considerably! Jesus said, "He who has My commandments and keeps them, he it is who loves Me" (John 14:21). To love God is to desire his glory above all things. Everything else becomes secondary. There may be times when the only *good* to come out of an experience is God's *glory*. If we truly love him, nothing else really matters. Knowing this will keep us from reading Romans 8:28 selfishly, as if everything that happens is ultimately intended for our good. It may well prove to be good for us, but only as a means by which we in turn become instruments for God's glory.

Having restricted the promise in this way, to those that love God, why does Paul go on to describe us as being the "called according to His purpose"? Paul apparently wants to make sure everyone understands that the only reason we love God is because he first loved us and graciously called us to himself. We are by nature prone to conclude that if God works all things together for good, it is because we have loved him, and he is simply rewarding us for the meritorious deed of loving him. May it never be! It is not because we love God that he causes all things to work together for good, but *because God first loved us* and called us according to his purpose.

Whatever your problem, whatever your pain, remember the promise of Paul. In *all* things, yes *all* things, God works marvelously and mysteriously for your good. Well indeed did the hymnwriter say:

> Fear not, I am with thee, O be not dismayed,
> For I am thy God, and will still give thee aid;
> I'll strengthen thee, help thee, and cause thee to stand,
> Upheld by My gracious omnipotent hand.

> When thro' the deep waters I call thee to go,
> The rivers of sorrow shall not overflow;
> For I will be with thee, thy trials to bless,
> And sanctify to thee thy deepest distress.

> When thro' fiery trials thy pathway shall lie,
> My grace, all sufficient shall be thy supply;
> The flames shall not hurt thee, I only design
> Thy dross to consume, and thy gold to refine.

The soul that on Jesus hath leaned for repose,
I will not, I will not, desert to his foes;
That soul, tho' all hell should endeavor to shake,
I'll never, no never, no never forsake!

Author unknown

14

"WHY ME, LORD?" OR, SUFFERING AND GOD'S PURPOSE

At the age of 29 John was the picture of health, as well as bright, articulate, and hardworking. Although no one would mistake him for Brooks Robinson, he played a pretty good third base on our church league softball team. He and his wife Nancy were the proud parents of a three-month-old baby girl. Above all else, John loved the Lord Jesus Christ and was growing mightily in grace and truth.

When I telephoned John to see if he wanted to play in the fall softball league, he declined. His back had been hurting him, he said, and he thought it might be better if he sat it out. Besides, Nancy needed help with the baby. One week later John was in an ambulance on his way to Dallas. The white blood count in a healthy person is 10,000. John's count had soared to 63,000. Leukemia.

As I stood at his bedside, I trembled. I couldn't believe this was the same man who only days before was laughing and working and playing with his new baby daughter. John was dying, and I wanted some answers. So did Nancy. We spent a long time talking about it and came away empty. We just didn't know why. But we knew that God did, and that was enough.

John survived those first few weeks. Chemotherapy took its toll on him, but in the providence of God it seemed to be working. As I sit writing this chapter, it has been about three months since the ordeal began. John is preparing to begin bone marrow transplants, and we are constantly in prayer for him. Nancy waits patiently. Little Kristen, now six months old, doesn't know what is happening. Some day she will, especially when she reads the letter her daddy found the strength to write one day as he lay wondering, "Why *me*, Lord?" The letter was addressed to our church.

Dear Christian Brothers,

After being awakened around 5:00 A.M. yesterday, the Lord began directing my thought towards writing this letter. Below are the messages that He wanted me to convey.

God's love, wisdom and power are so enormous that our feeble minds can only begin to comprehend it all. It is therefore so critical that we Christians place *every* aspect of our *entire* lives *totally* in the hands of God. God will not let us down and will never give us more than we can handle. He loves us so much and has a plan for us all.

So do not despair for me. Our Father is in total control. But please continue your prayers for me, which are being answered. Your prayers and notes have been a great source of strength and inspiration throughout this mission which the Lord has sent me on.

The power of prayer is immeasurable. God can and does work miracles through prayer. Using my doctors, I am convinced God is working a miracle for me now. My doctors seem baffled at how well I have progressed this past week. Praise the Lord!

In Christ's name, I love you all,

John

I felt so small when I read that. You see, I argue with God about minor inconveniences. I tend to run out of patience over the trifles of life. I complain about insignificant burdens that I must bear. John, on the other hand, could only see his fight with leukemia as a mission. A mission! Boy, I feel small!

All of us have suffered at some time in our lives, some more than others. We all know what it means to hurt. Then there are those, like John, whom God decides to send on a mission. I'm not talking about the minor irritations of life. I'm talking about leukemia before you're 30, diabetes, the death of a child, multiple sclerosis, paralysis. These are the afflictions that really challenge a person's faith, that really test one's trust.

The world has a quick fix for this sort of suffering. Its advice is simple: Curse God and die! The charade is over. Admit that it was all a delusion and face the facts—if God really loved you, he wouldn't let you suffer in this way. But the child of God knows better. John knows better. That is why his letter speaks so confidently of God's love and sovereignty. That isn't to say his pain is any less intense or real. But he knows in his heart that it isn't a charade. He knows that God really does love him.

So why do God's people suffer? That's what this chapter is all about. But don't expect any easy answers. There aren't any. Glib, complacent explanations of why God's people suffer don't do anybody any good, least of all those who are suffering. What we need are caring, sensitive and, above all, *biblical* answers to life's tough questions. Of course, the answers have always been there. It isn't as though we are discovering them for the first time. I won't pretend to say anything truly original or profound in this chapter. Our problem is not with finding answers but with accepting them. God has already told us the reasons his people suffer. The rub is that we don't always like what he says. It takes time. Nobody learns these lessons overnight. In her book *A Step Further*, Joni Eareckson Tada describes her own struggle.

> But today as I look back, I am convinced that the whole ordeal of my paralysis was inspired by His love. I wasn't a rat in a maze. I wasn't the brunt of some cruel divine joke. God had *reasons* behind my suffering, and learning some of them has made all the difference in the world. He has reasons for your suffering, too.[1]

No, contrary to what you may be thinking, that *wasn't* easy for her to say. In fact, the only way she could say it was with a pencil held tightly in her teeth. If anyone knows suffering, she does. I'll be the first to confess I'm no Job. But Joni knows whereof she speaks. So if you won't believe me, believe her: God does have reasons for your suffering. Let me mention five of them.

To Conform Us to Christ's Image
We may readily acknowledge that the goal of Christian experience is conformity to the image of Christ. Paul makes this clear

enough in several places (cf. Rom. 8:29). But we are not as quick to accept that many Christ-like qualities come only through suffering. My sinful nature is to wish it were not so, but it is. Paul says it plainly in Romans 5:3-5. "And not only this, but we also exult in our tribulations, knowing that tribulation brings about perseverance; and perseverance, proven character; and proven character, hope; and hope does not disappoint, because the love of God has been poured out within our hearts through the Holy Spirit who was given to us." James agrees. "Consider it all joy, my brethren, when you encounter various trials, knowing that the testing of your faith produces endurance. And let endurance have its perfect result, that you may be perfect and complete, lacking in nothing (James 1:2-4; cf. 1 Pet. 1:6-9).

I have always been amazed by the skills of the sculptor. Although I have only seen Michelangelo's *David* in a picture, it baffles me how any man could produce something so striking and lifelike. Someone once said that sculpting is easy: you just chip away everything that doesn't look like a man! When I read passages such as those by Paul and James and Peter, it is as if they envision God to be a sculptor of sorts, with our trials and pains the hammer and chisel used to shape us into the image of Christ. All he does is chip away from our lives everything that doesn't look like Jesus!

Christian virtues like faith, patience, endurance, and dependence on God often come at a high price—our pain. "When you crush lavender," wrote David Watson, shortly before his death, "you find its full fragrance; when you squeeze an orange, you extract its sweet juice. In the same way it is often through pains and hurts that we develop the fragrance and sweetness of Jesus in our lives."[2]

To Prepare Us for Ministry

Sometimes we suffer because God wants us to minister to others, sometimes because God wants others to minister to us. In other words, suffering is what binds believers together. God is glorified when his children display Christ-like compassion and tenderness one to another. As Joni has said, "One of God's purposes in increasing our trials is to sensitize us to people we never would have been able to relate to otherwise."[3] This is what Paul is saying in 2 Corinthians 1:3-7. There he describes a marvelous "cycle of comfort" that brings Christians into touch with one another.

> Praise be to the God and Father of our Lord Jesus Christ, the Father of compassion and the God of all comfort, who comforts us in all our troubles, so that we can comfort those in any trouble with the comfort we ourselves have received from God. For just as the sufferings of Christ flow over into our lives, so also through Christ our comfort overflows. If we are distressed, it is for your comfort and salvation; if we are comforted, it is for your comfort, which produces in you patient endurance of the same sufferings we suffer. And our hope for you is firm, because we know that just as you share in our sufferings, so also you share in our comfort (NIV).

This is one reason I am convinced that the gospel of health and wealth being preached today is fundamentally *selfish*. It is oriented to *me* and what *I* need and can obtain from God. But affliction, whatever its form, is really God's way of preparing us to minister to others. Without it the body of Christ would be largely deprived of the deep feelings of mutual dependence and love. So when you are hurting, don't ask, "Why *me*, Lord?" Ask "Who *else*, Lord?" For God may well have permitted your pain in order that he might channel his comfort through you to others who are in need.

To Provide Us Opportunities for Witness

We can witness to the lost in many ways, but rarely can we do so more effectively than when we suffer. For when we praise God in the midst of our afflictions, it shows the world how great and majestic he must be to inspire such loyalty in his children.

Charles Colson has given us a stirring account of his own bout with cancer and what he learned from it. In particular he describes the opportunity it provided him to share his faith, an opportunity he might otherwise never have had. (Reprinted from *Christianity Today* © 1987. Used by permission of Prison Fellowship Ministries, P.O. Box 17500, Washington, DC 20041.)

During my nightly walks through the hospital corridors, dragging an IV pole behind me, I often met an Indian man whose two-year-old son had had two failed kidney transplants, a brain aneurysm, and was now blind for life.

When the father, a Hindu, discovered I was a Christian, he asked if God would heal his son if he, too, was born again. He said he had heard things like that on television.

As I listened, I realized how arrogant health-and-wealth religion sounds to suffering families: Christians can all be spared suffering, but little Hindu children go blind. One couldn't blame a Hindu or Muslim or agnostic for resenting, even hating, such a God.

I told my Hindu friend about Jesus. Yes, he may miraculously intervene in our lives. But we come to God not because of what he may do to spare us suffering, but because Christ is truth. What he does promise us is much more—the forgiveness of sin and eternal life. I left the hospital with my friend studying Christian literature, the Bible, and my own account in *Born Again*. If he becomes a Christian, it won't be on false pretenses.

I thought often in the hospital of the words of Florida pastor Steve Brown. Steve says that every time a non-Christian gets cancer, God allows a Christian to get cancer as well—so the world can see the difference. I prayed I might be so filled with God's grace that the world might see the difference.

Steve's words represent a powerful truth. God does not witness to the world by taking his people out of suffering, but rather by demonstrating his grace through them in the midst of pain.

He allows such weakness to reveal his strength in adversity. His own Son experienced brokenness—and died—that we might be freed from the power of death. But we are promised no freedom from suffering until we are beyond the grave.

Thus, I can only believe that God allowed my cancer for a purpose—just as he allows far more horrific and deadly cancers in fellow Christians every day. We don't begin to know all the reasons why. But we do know that our suffering and weakness can be an opportunity to witness to the world the amazing grace of God at work through us.[4]

To Awaken Us to Divine Grace

One of the most subtle and vicious of human sins is presumption. We take for granted so very much, not thinking of the price that often must be paid for our privileges. We talk about our "rights" as if God owed us something, when in fact it only took one sin for us to forfeit the right to life itself. We breathe and live and love and laugh only because God is long-suffering and gracious. Yet we presume upon his grace, thinking that God is indebted to us. That is why we get so upset when we suffer. Our problem is that we actually believe we *deserve* pleasure and good health. But all we have ever deserved is death and condemnation. That's what makes grace so gracious!

Suffering is one of God's ways of getting our attention in order to remind us that everything we have is of grace. Our sinful inclination is to forget about God when things are going well. C. S. Lewis put it best in what is perhaps his most famous saying: "God whispers to us in our pleasures . . . but shouts in our pains: it is His megaphone to rouse a deaf world."[5] Joni says much the same thing. "During my stay in the hospital," she writes, "I met many people who wouldn't have given God the time of day when they were healthy. But a good splash of ice-cold suffering sure woke them out of their spiritual slumber."[6]

Sometimes there just isn't any other way to wean us from ourselves except by making us hurt. That isn't God's fault. It is *our* fault. Suffering is God's way of bringing us back in touch with himself and his grace. It is his way of shaking the cobwebs of self-sufficiency and pride from our hearts. Health and wealth, though they may be divine blessings, are all too often distorted into excuses for ignoring God. But pain dramatizes our need for him. It keeps us from relegating God to little more than a footnote in our lives. Let us never forget that the most grievous disease is not bodily affliction, but the loss of spiritual intimacy with God. Suffering drives us to our knees, thrusts us before the throne of grace, and welds us to the heart of our heavenly Father.

To Show Us God's Glory

Of all things Joni Eareckson Tada has written about suffering, the following statement is easily the most remarkable.

> I sometimes shudder to think where I would be today if I had
> not broken my neck. I couldn't see at first why God would
> possibly allow it, but I sure do now. He has gotten so much
> more glory through my paralysis than through my health!
> And believe me, you'll never know how rich that makes me
> feel.[7]

She is right. I probably never will know, unless God should send
similar suffering my way. Though it has come at a high price, Joni
has learned the ultimate reason for human existence—God's glory.
The Protestant Reformers of the sixteenth century had a Latin
phrase for it: *Soli Deo Gloria*, "Glory to God Only!" Joni now
knows in a way she never knew before that God doesn't exist for
her; rather, she exists for God. And how *rich* it makes her feel. Not
bitter or resentful or angry, but *rich!*

Although David Watson did not share Joni's theological perspective on divine healing, he certainly agreed with her on this vital
truth. In *Fear No Evil* he wrote these moving words:

> The sparkling radiance of a diamond is caused by a lump of
> coal subjected to extreme pressure and heat over a long period
> of time. Again a beautiful pearl emerges when an oyster has to
> cover an irritating object with layer upon layer of smooth
> mother-of-pearl lining excreted from its own body. When we
> suffer in various ways, God is able to use all the pressures and
> irritations to reveal something of his radiance and beauty in
> our lives.[8]

At issue is our willingness to be instruments for God's glory. If we
are not willing, whatever the cost, then suffering will remain a puzzle to us, an enigma, an ever-threatening obstacle to our growth in
grace. No one ever said it was easy—at least no one who ever truly
suffered. But I'm convinced the above perspective on suffering is
true because it is biblical. May God help us to write across all our
pains: SOLI DEO GLORIA!

Did God ever heal John? Yes, in a manner of speaking he did.
On February 13, 1988, God healed him into heaven.

ADDENDUM
PERSECUTION AND PAIN

Some charismatics have attempted to evade the implications of what I have just said by distinguishing between the suffering caused by persecution and the suffering caused by disease. They realize there are too many personal examples and explicit statements in the Bible to deny that God permits his people to suffer. So they concede that persecution and oppression are within God's will for believers. We can expect to be deprived, abused, slandered, perhaps beaten or even martyred by the world. But such physical persecution, we are told, is not the same thing as physical sickness. The latter is *not* within God's will for the believer. Thus Francis MacNutt makes a distinction between persecution, or suffering that comes "*from outside* a man because of the wickedness of other men who are evil," and sickness, "the suffering that tears man apart *from within*, whether it be physical, emotional, or moral."[9]

And so some charismatics would have us believe that when the apostle Paul in 2 Corinthians 12:10 refers to "weakness," "insults," "distresses," "persecutions," and "difficulties," he does not mean bodily illnesses. Instead, these experiences, with which Paul is "well content," are the effects of anti-Christian hostility, not viruses or tumors or destructive organisms. God may will that you suffer, but he never wills that you suffer from sickness.

Is that a valid distinction, and if so, is it significant in terms of our discussion? The answer to the first question is yes; the answer to the second is no. The distinction, though perhaps technically valid, centers merely on the cause of suffering, not its nature.

Let me illustrate. Suppose that in the course of his apostolic ministry the apostle Paul is stoned by Jewish antagonists and suffers a broken and subsequently deformed hand as a result. The hand receives severe nerve and structural damage and is basically useless to Paul. Silas, Paul's companion, is also stoned but escapes serious injury. Nevertheless, he also has a hand that is of little use to him because of advanced rheumatoid arthritis. Both men suffer, through no fault of their own. Both have lost the use of a hand.

What would the charismatic have us say to them? Should we tell Silas that God is *not* willing for his hand to hurt and that he wills to heal him? Or should we tell Paul that God *is* willing for his hand to hurt and that he most likely will *not* heal him? Does God say to Silas, "Since your pain is caused by some biological enemy within you, I will heal it" but to Paul, "Because your pain is caused by some human enemy outside you I will *not* heal it"? If God is willing to heal Silas, why not Paul also? Both of their afflictions may deter them in their evangelistic duties. Why should God consider Paul's disability permissible, but not Silas's?

If there is healing for the body in the atonement, healing we may always experience now, why should Paul have to suffer any more than Silas? The bottom line in both cases is that the human body is a frail, susceptible, corruptible vessel. If part of Christ's redemptive work on the cross was to guarantee healing and deliverance for the body now (as the charismatic insists), what reasonable difference does it make whether pain is caused by a biological organism or an anti-Christian mob?

The implication of this is clear and unmistakable. If what the charismatic says about God's will for physical health and wholeness is true, I don't see how God can will *any* suffering. But of course we know that he does, a fact even the charismatic Christian is forced to admit. If God does will that the righteous suffer from persecution, there is no reasonable way to deny that he wills they suffer from sickness. Bodily suffering is bodily suffering, irrespective of its cause. If God is willing to permit it in the one case, he must be willing to permit it in the other.

EPILOGUE

John Calvin is one of the most misunderstood men in the history of the Christian church. The mere mention of his name conjures up in many the image of a stern, Scrooge-like figure who kicked puppies, burned heretics, and smiled with a sadistic glee in his eyes whenever he heard the word "hell." Those responsible for such slander and misrepresentation must answer to God for their lies. John Calvin, quite simply, was one of the kindest, most generous, self-sacrificing, and, yes, brilliant Christian men who ever lived. His is a fascinating story. But more important for our purposes, it is instructive and inspiring as well. For we see in Calvin and his struggle with suffering what I believe God expects from each of us.

Calvin's Life and Labors

Calvin was born on July 10, 1509, at Noyon in northeastern France. His father was wealthy enough to provide John with an excellent education. After receiving his A.B. degree from the University of Paris in 1528, he studied law at the University of Orleans and later returned to Paris to study the classics.

No one is certain when Calvin was converted to faith in Christ, but most think it was sometime in 1531. He was saved not out of immoral paganism, but out of the legalism of the Roman Catholic Church, to which he had been fervently devoted. "God himself produced the change," he wrote. "When I was obstinately addicted to the superstitions of the papacy, God subdued and reduced my heart to docility." Again, "only one haven of salvation is left open for our souls, and that is the mercy of God in Christ. We are saved by grace—not by our merits, not by our works."

Calvin's new life in Christ and belief in salvation by the sovereignty of divine grace alone transformed an old friend, the Roman Catholic Church, into a new enemy. Late in 1533 he was forced to flee Paris much as the apostle Paul fled Damascus. He was let down from a window by means of sheets tied together and escaped from the city disguised as a vine-dresser with a hoe upon his shoulder. He spent the next two years as a wandering student and evangelist.

He finally settled in Basel, Switzerland, and began what he hoped would be a life-long career as a scholar and author. But as he later explained, "God thrust me into the game!" It was during his stay in Basel that Calvin began work on what was to become (in my opinion) the greatest work of Christian theology ever written (other than Holy Scripture itself). *The Institutes of the Christian Religion* appeared in its first edition in March of 1536. Calvin became famous overnight.

One must understand that Calvin wished not to become directly involved in the Protestant Reformation, except by way of writing in its defense. He did not envision himself a strong man who, like Martin Luther, could stand up to the hostility of the papacy. But God had other plans, and only the blind can fail to see divine providence in the turn of events that brought Calvin to Geneva.

As he was making his way to Strasbourg, he was detoured to Geneva because of the war raging between Francis I and Charles V. He planned only to stay that one night and then continue his journey. But William Farel, a man who labored long and hard for the Reformation in Geneva, received word that Calvin was in town. The encounter that ensued is one of the most dramatic and historically significant events in the history of the church.

"You are not leaving, that's off!" shouted Farel. "There is much for you to do here."

"What do you mean?" asked Calvin. "I am sorry, but I cannot remain any longer than one night."

Farel paid no attention. With great eloquence he described the miraculous work of God in the city of Geneva and the need for a man of Calvin's stature and skill to come to teach. Calvin protested, expressing his desire to spend his time writing in the safety of some remote city.

"Leisure, learning—when it is a matter of acting!" shouted Farel in indignation. "Do you want to desert the Reformation of this city? I am at the point of breaking down under the load and you will deny me your assistance!"

"Don't take it as ill-will," said Calvin. "My health is not the best; I need a rest."

"What rest!" cried Farel. "Nothing except death brings rest to the servants of Christ! Do you dare put your personal interests ahead of the kingdom of God?"

Calvin quivered. The reproach of putting his personal comfort ahead of the service of Christ caused him severe qualms of conscience. The storm had begun in Calvin's soul, as the two men wrangled throughout the night. Farel was determined to break his resistance. Forgetting all formality, Farel shouted: "For the last time, do you want to follow the call of God, or don't you?"

"No! No! No!" shouted Calvin.

Farel's stature became erect; his eyes hurled lightning. "You are concerned about your rest and your personal interests. Therefore, I proclaim to you in the name of Almighty God whose command you defy: Upon your work there shall rest no blessing! Therefore, let God damn your rest, let God damn your work!"

Wide-eyed, Calvin stared at the small lips which had pronounced this horrible curse. He trembled as it all suddenly became clear to him. Farel was only an instrument, a vessel through whom the Lord himself was speaking. A feeling overtook him as bitter as death. He saw himself suddenly torn out of the path which had opened up before him, and found himself stationed in battle and unrest—in the front line. As if under searing fire, Calvin's defiance melted. And as he offered his hand to the preacher, a tear rolled over his caved-in cheek. "I obey God!" was his cry.[1]

Upon his arrival in Geneva Calvin immediately went to work, lecturing on the Pauline epistles, writing a constitution for the church, introducing congregational psalm singing, writing a confession of faith and a children's catechism, and insisting on the frequent observance of the Lord's Supper.

Both Calvin and Farel faced resistance from the beginning. Their efforts to administer discipline both within and outside the church met with stiff opposition. Eventually they were both kicked out of town. Calvin spent a brief time in Basel before settling in Strasbourg, where he remained from May of 1538 until September of 1541.

While in Strasbourg Calvin decided to look for a wife. He said he didn't care what she looked like as long as she could take care of him, was of a Christian spirit, and could interact with him intellectually (no small consideration!). Farel tried to set him up with one young lady, but the relationship came to a quick and decisive end when Calvin insisted that she first learn to speak French. He finally married Idelette de Bure in 1540, who had two children from a previous marriage. She died in 1549. All three of their children died young.

In the meantime the situation in Geneva had worsened. Forces friendly to Calvin and Farel regained power and convinced him to return. Although Calvin was given a free hand to bring the Reformation to Geneva, he faced opposition from several fronts. One thing that aroused the ire of many was his insistence that only believers should be admitted to partake of the Lord's Supper. Interestingly, two centuries later Jonathan Edwards faced the same problem in colonial America. Edwards was eventually thrown out of his own church for refusing to permit unbelievers to sit at communion. Calvin, however, survived. He employed strict measures of examination to be certain those partaking of the elements were truly Christians. On one occasion a group of citizens who had been refused the Supper armed themselves and entered the church, seeking to force their admission to communion. They threatened Calvin's life if he did not serve them the bread and the wine. When he spread his hands out over the elements and declared that they would partake over his dead body, they withdrew.

Calvin's success in bringing the Reformation to Geneva was due in no small part to his almost super-human endurance and dedication to the Lord Jesus Christ. His normal practice was to preach twice on Sunday and on each day of the week, every other week. This was in addition to his theological lectures, his pastoral duties, his writing ministry, and his indefatigable efforts on behalf of the city itself.

There were, however, several problems in his family that brought Calvin great personal sorrow and exposed him unfairly to public ridicule. The wife of his brother Antoine was caught in adultery, but was found innocent. Later, she was again caught, this time with Calvin's own house servant. This same servant, whom Calvin trusted implicitly, was discovered to have been stealing from Calvin for years. Then his step-daughter was also caught in adultery. He often remarked that nothing in his life was more grievous to his heart than these moral indiscretions by those close to him.

It is impossible to describe fully the labors of John Calvin on behalf of the kingdom of God. Perhaps no one before or since in the history of the church has expended himself more diligently for the cause of Christ. There were no limits to which he would not go in the interests of godliness. It comes as little surprise to those who know of his efforts that his influence on the development of the Christian church in the Western world is immeasurable.[2]

Calvin's Ill Health

Why have I taken the time to chronicle the life and labors of John Calvin? What possible relevance does he have for our study of divine healing? Very simply this: John Calvin was a physical wreck. His holiness has never been in question, and yet his health was an unmitigated disaster. Throughout his professional and ministerial career he was plagued with countless maladies. A lesser man would have become bitter and resentful, perhaps even despondent of God's love. Not John Calvin.

His afflictions read like a medical journal. He suffered from painful stomach cramps, intestinal influenza, and recurring migraine headaches. He was subject to a persistent onslaught of fevers that would often lay him up for weeks at a time. He experienced problems with his trachea, in addition to pleurisy, gout, and colic. He was especially susceptible to hemorrhoids, which were aggravated by an internal abscess that would not heal. He suffered from severe arthritis and acute pain in his knees, calves, and feet. Other maladies included nephritis (acute, chronic inflammation of the kidney caused by infection), gallstones, and kidney stones. He once passed a kidney stone so large that it tore the urinary canal and led to excessive bleeding.

One of the most problematic of his many afflictions resulted from his rigorous preaching schedule. He would often strain his voice so severely that he experienced violent fits of coughing. On one occasion he broke a blood-vessel in his lungs and hemorrhaged. When he reached the age of 51, it was discovered that he was suffering from pulmonary tuberculosis, which would ultimately prove fatal. Much of his study and writing he carried on while bedridden. In the final few years of his life he had to be carried to work.

His friends frequently urged him to ease off the demanding pace he had set for himself. When told by his physicians that he simply must rest, he responded: "What! Would you have the Lord find me idle when he comes?" Calvin preached his last sermon on February 6, 1564. He had to be carried to and from the pulpit. He dictated his will on April 25th. It read, in part, as follows:

> In the name of God, I John Calvin, servant of the Word of God in the Church of Geneva, weakened by many illnesses . . . thank God that He has shown not only his mercy toward me, His poor creature, and . . . has suffered me in all sins and weaknesses, but what is more, that He has made me a partaker of His grace to serve Him through my work, . . . I confess to live and die in this faith which He has given me, inasmuch as I have no other hope or refuge than His predestination upon which my entire salvation is grounded. I embrace the grace which He has offered me in our Lord Jesus Christ and accept the merits of His suffering and dying that through them all my sins are buried.

I don't know what today's faith healers think of John Calvin. Perhaps they would prefer not to think of him at all. But I cannot help thinking of him often. I think of him whenever I hurt and am inclined to complain. I think of him when others say God never wills that his people should suffer. I think of him when the uninformed callously suggest that illness is the effect of an insufficient faith.

Someone may argue that if Calvin achieved so much in spite of his afflictions, imagine what he might have done without them. But I am not so sure. I am more inclined to believe that he accomplished what he did precisely because his illnesses compelled him to rely on the sufficiency of divine grace in a way he otherwise never would have. His pain drove him to the comfort that only God can supply. His weakness compelled him to seek the divine truth that Paul and Joni Eareckson Tada and others like them have found only in Christ. No, I am not saying that it is bad to be healthy. God forbid. But neither is it necessarily bad to be afflicted. For when we are weak, then he is strong.

Calvin's coat of arms, a hand holding a heart, is testimony to his compassionate and self-sacrificial spirit. It is encircled by his motto: *Cor meum tibi offero Domine prompte et sincere.* Freely translated it means, "My heart for Thy cause I offer Thee, Lord, promptly and sincerely." My guess is he probably wrote that in pain.

APPENDIX A

THE DEFEAT OF THE DEVIL

Not too long ago I came across an interesting cartoon in which two people are exiting a movie theater. In the background several posters and a marquis suggest that they have recently viewed one of the many so-called "devil" pictures so prominent today. The one person turns to the other and says: "Oh, I believe in the supernatural. I just don't believe in God."

While many people are humored by that sort of reaction, few are surprised by it. One need only look to Hollywood to understand why. In the past two decades Americans have been subjected to a virtual flood of "cinematic devilmania." It all started with *Rosemary's Baby*, after which came *The Exorcist*, its sequel *The Heretic*, *Omen I* and *Omen II*, *The Amityville Horror*, *Poltergeist I* and *II*, and *Ghostbusters*. Little wonder that people have come to believe in the existence and power of the devil and his demonic hosts while paying only lip service to the divine side of the supernatural.

Contributing to this trend is the way Hollywood usually portrays the devil and his cohorts as more powerful and cunning than anything or anyone that traditional religion can bring to bear against them. I am reminded particularly of *The Exorcist*, in which the demon is able to resist the power of the clergy at length and eventually cause the death of a Roman Catholic priest. That kind of story line may make for successful cinematic theatrics, but it is utterly contrary to the biblical gospel. Hollywood scriptwriters could do with a healthy dose of 1 John 4:4, where the apostle reminds his Christian readers that "greater is He who is in you than he who is in the world."

What makes this especially disheartening is that many Christians today have lost sight of this glorious truth and behave as if

Satan were more powerful than the Son of God! It is a sad day
when professing believers fear Satan more than they trust the Son;
when the comfort of Christ's gracious presence receives less attention than the prospect of demonic activity; when prayer in times of
trouble is displaced by a fascination with binding and denouncing
the devil; when instead of drawing on the power of the Holy Spirit
to overcome the temptations of the flesh, believers shift blame for
every sin (and affliction) onto some demon from which they are
convinced they need to be delivered.

I am persuaded that much of this is due to the failure of Christians to understand and appreciate that the decisive battle between God and the forces of evil has already been fought and won!
Contrary to what one popular author would have us believe,
Satan is *not* alive and well on planet earth! He is alive, but not
well. He has received a deadly blow, his judgment has come, his
doom is sealed. Though he still prowls about as a roaring lion seeking whom he may devour (1 Pet. 5:8), his authority and power have
been checked, and his days are numbered (cf. Rev. 12:12). Because
of what our Lord Jesus has accomplished by his death, resurrection, and exaltation, we have the promise that if we resist the
devil, he *will* flee from us (James 4:7; 1 Pet. 5:9). Yes, we are engaged
in a spiritual war (Eph. 6:10-20). But it is a war the outcome of
which has already been decided in our favor! We fight against a defeated foe, over whom we have complete authority and from
whom we need fear nothing. He has been arrested, convicted, and
sentenced to imprisonment and is but for the moment free on bail
(cf. Matt. 25:41; 1 Cor. 15:24-28; Rev. 20:7-10).

The devil was crushed for the first time by our Lord when he
tried but failed to seduce the Savior in the wilderness. Wielding
the Word of God, Jesus resisted the temptations of Satan and
thereby proved himself an altogether adequate high priest, who is
able to intercede on our behalf and aid us in our own fight against
Satanic solicitation (cf. Matt. 4:1-11; Heb. 2:17-18; 4:15). Time and
again Jesus cast out demons, demonstrating both his power over
the devil and the presence of the kingdom (cf. Matt. 12:22-29). In
anticipation of his cross-work, Jesus declared, "Now judgment is
upon this world; now the ruler of this world shall be cast out"

(John 12:31; cf. 16:11). The apostle John tells us that "the Son of God appeared for this purpose, that He might destroy the works of the devil" (1 John 3:8). And that is precisely what he did. The author of the epistle to the Hebrews speaks of how Jesus partook of flesh and blood "that through death He might render powerless him who had the power of death, that is, the devil; and might deliver those who through fear of death were subject to slavery all their lives" (Heb. 2:14-15).

Perhaps the most graphic and instructive statement concerning the defeat of the devil is found in Colossians 2:15. God the Father, through God the Son, has "disarmed the rulers and authorities," and has "made a public display of them, having triumphed over them through Him." The "rulers and authorities" or "principalities and powers" are undoubtedly the devil and his demonic hordes (cf. Eph. 1:20-21; 3:10; 6:10ff.; Rom. 8:38).[1] Paul says that Christ has "disarmed" them. This is the same verb he uses later in Colossians 3:9 when he urges believers to "lay aside" or to "strip themselves" of sin as if it were a filthy garment.

We all remember the story of Hercules in ancient mythology. It is said that on one occasion Hercules was travelling with his wife Deianira when they came upon a flooded stream. He permitted a centaur named Nessus to carry Deianira across the waters, only to shoot him with a poisonous arrow when Nessus was rude to her. As the centaur lay dying, he told Deianira to save his blood as a love charm. Later, when Hercules fell in love with Iole, Deianira dipped a rope in the blood of Nessus and sent it to her husband. When he put it on, poison began to eat away his flesh. In agony, this once mighty man of mythology begged his friends to burn his body and put an end to his painful ordeal.

This story provided Bishop J. B. Lightfoot with just the illustration he needed to drive home the point of Paul's statement in Colossians 2:15. "The powers of evil," he explained, "which had clung like a Nessus robe about His [Christ's] humanity, were torn off and cast aside forever."[2] The forces of the devil and darkness had beset our Lord at every turn of his earthly life and ministry. He was, as it were, enshrouded by their poisonous hostility, subject to their persistent assault. But unlike the mythological Hercules, whose death was his defeat, our Lord triumphed over his foes through the cross. In his crucifixion he stripped the forces of evil from himself as one would an old and filthy garment.

But that is not all. He also made a public display of the demonic hosts, exposing them to ridicule by triumphing over them through that very instrument by which they thought he was defeated. Note that the final phrase in Colossians 2:15 should be translated "having triumphed over them through *it*," that is, through the *Cross*! The tree that to every eye appeared to be the cause of his demise became the tool of his triumph. In a marvelous twist of divine irony, the instrument of disgrace and death by which the devil thought he had gained victory became the weapon of his own destruction.

The reality and finality of Christ's defeat of the devil was confirmed when God raised him from the dead and exalted him to the right hand of the majesty on high (cf. Eph. 1:20-23; Rev. 1:17-18; 12:1-17). It is because Jesus is Lord, the Ruler and King of all rulers and kings, that we are assured of victory over the forces of evil.

Let us go forth to battle, therefore, with the words of Martin Luther on our lips:

> And tho' this world, with devils filled,
> Should threaten to undo us;
> We will not fear, for God hath willed
> His truth to triumph through us.
> The prince of darkness grim —
> We tremble not for him;
> His rage we can endure,
> For lo! his doom is sure,
> One little word shall fell him.

APPENDIX B

WAS JESUS EVER SICK?

It is sometimes said that Christians should not be sick because Christ never was. Writes Colin Urquhart:

> Jesus lived in perfect "wholeness"; He neither sinned nor was He ever sick. In one sense we all need healing because none of us is yet perfect like Him. Sickness is a failure to be like Jesus. He was the man who lived human life to the full. He was never sick because He never sinned; He never became tainted with the fallen nature of creation.[1]

Several comments are in order. First, the New Testament is silent on whether Jesus was ever sick. While it never records an occasion on which Jesus was ill, we may not deduce from silence that he never was. The Bible makes no statement either way. Why, then, are charismatic authors such as Urquhart and MacNutt so dogmatic on this issue? Because they either *identify* sickness with sin or argue that all sickness is the *result* of sin. Urquhart says that "sickness is a failure to be like Jesus" and that Jesus "was never sick because He never sinned." But as I pointed out in chapter 2, sickness per se is not sin—we are never told to repent of the flu or to confess asthma or to feel guilty for arthritis. Certainly Jesus never sinned. But Urquhart's inference that he was never sick assumes a false theological premise—that sickness is always directly tied to some specific sin (cf. chapter 6, as well as Jesus' own statement in John 9:1-3).

Urquhart also says that Jesus "never became tainted with the fallen nature of creation." If by this he means that the human nature of Jesus was not sinful flesh, I agree (see Rom. 8:3). But if he means that Jesus' human nature was invulnerable to illness, I must demur. The New Testament is clear that Jesus assumed a human nature like ours in every respect, except sin (see Heb. 2:14-18; 4:15; 1 John 4:2). Because he was a man, Jesus was open to temptation. But because he was God, it was impossible that he should succumb to it.

However, Jesus' freedom from sin does not imply that he was free from the mishaps and miscalculations that are an inevitable part of living in a fallen world. For example, I'm sure that while working in his father's carpentry shop Jesus at some time hit his thumb with a hammer. And when he did, he probably yelled "Ouch!" (or whatever they yelled in that culture—short of profanity). I also believe that because of his human nature, Jesus had to learn to read and write, and subtract, and multiply and divide just as other children did. In doing so he undoubtedly made mistakes.

But missing a nail and hitting one's thumb is not a sin. It is a *physical* lapse, not a *moral* one. And thinking that $5 \times 5 = 30$, when first learning the multiplication tables, is not a sin. It is a mental mistake, not a moral transgression. No moral law of God is deliberately or even inadvertently violated in these cases. Such mishaps and mistakes are only to be expected of anyone who lives in a fallen, imperfect world.

We can be sure that Jesus never dishonored his parents, never cheated at games with his playmates, never stole an apple from a neighbor's tree, never cursed his fellow man (or God). And yet, if given a rotten apple by his neighbor, he would have suffered a stomach ache upon eating it. Jesus thirsted, but never lusted; hungered, but never lied; experienced pain but never impurity. If hit, he bled, but never retaliated. So let us remember that because he was human, he was in all things like us, but because he was God, he was without sin or moral fault.[2]

Imagine for a moment. Would Jesus ever have had a headache from the hot summer sun in Palestine? Might he have suffered from allergies? Might he ever have experienced stomach problems from drinking impure water? If he struck his thumb in the carpentry shop, would it have swollen up and turned black and blue, or perhaps have become infected? These are not silly questions. When the second person of the Trinity took to himself human flesh, a human nature, he became susceptible to all the experiences and ill-effects that come from living in a sinful world. Bodily illness and injury were no more contrary to the moral character of Jesus than intellectual ignorance (Mark 13:32) was contrary to his deity. Physical vulnerability was part of what it meant to be "in the form of a bond servant," "made in the likeness of men," and "found in appearance as a man" (Phil. 2:7-8).

No, I cannot *prove* that Jesus was ever ill, anymore than someone else can prove he was not. But if his body was of like nature with ours, he would have been exposed to the same organisms and viruses and bacteria that commonly attack us. He felt pain, he ran short of oxygen and tired, he bled when beaten and pierced, and he died physically. His body succumbed to the abuse of his executioners in the same way as did the bodies of the two thieves crucified with him.

It would seem, therefore, that the only reason for insisting that Jesus was never sick is that Jesus never sinned. But this is itself based on the ill-founded assumption that if one does not sin, one will not get sick, and, if one is sick it is because one has sinned. Perhaps when we get to heaven, we shall discover that Jesus was never ill. But I doubt it.

APPENDIX C

A REVIEW OF JAMES RANDI'S THE FAITH-HEALERS

James Randi's *The Faith-Healers* (Buffalo: Prometheus, 1987) is a provocative book. Some will be provoked to praise it, while others will simply be provoked. In either case it is certainly worthy of our careful consideration.

The author, known professionally as "The Amazing Randi," is an accomplished magician who has appeared frequently in recent years on national television. I first saw him on the CBS news magazine show, "West 57th Street," when he exposed TV evangelist and faith healer Peter Popoff. He had earlier appeared on "The Tonight Show" with Johnny Carson, where he first announced his investigation of Popoff and other faith healers. Three weeks before I wrote this review of his book, he was a guest of talk show host Larry King on CNN, together with Marjoe Gortner and Reverend Ike.

Randi's Message

By his own confession James Randi is an angry man. His book, so he says, "is a cry of outrage against a wrong that needs to be righted" (5). It is fair to say that Randi is on something of a crusade. His target is what he considers a massive, nationwide scam among so-called faith healers. Randi is persuaded that "people are being robbed of their money, their health, and their emotional stability" (5) by a host of religious frauds. For the past several years he and a team of research assistants have devoted themselves to investigating claims of divine healing. *The Faith-Healers* is an account of his efforts to find *one* example of a healing that can stand rigorous scientific and medical examination. He insists that he has found none.

Several well-known faith healers are the unfortunate targets of Randi's rage. He devotes separate, probing chapters to A. A. Allen (one of the founding fathers of the modern healing movement; now deceased), Leroy Jenkins, W. V. Grant, Peter Popoff, Oral Roberts, Pat Robertson, Reverend Willard Fuller, Grace DiBiccari (also known as "Amazing Grace"), and Father DiOrio. Among the "lesser lights" whom Randi examines are Danny Davis, Kathryn Kuhlman, Daniel Atwood, David Epley, Brother Al Warick, David Paul, Ernest Angley, and The Happy Hunters.

There is no mistaking Randi's feelings about faith healing. He says that it is "difficult to differentiate from witchcraft, which in its healing aspects is involved with expelling evil spirits from the body" (32). Elsewhere he argues that "reduced to its basics, faith-healing today—as it always has been—is simply 'magic.' Though the preachers vehemently deny any connection with the practice, their activities meet all the requirements for the definition. All of the elements are present, and the intent is identical" (35). According to Randi, faith healing is flimflam, pure and simple. It differs little from real-estate schemes, vitamin frauds, and get-rich-quick hoaxes. He places faith healing in company with the bizarre special effects of an Alice Cooper rock concert and the well-orchestrated but obvious fakery of professional wrestling!

In a brief survey of the origins of faith healing Randi devotes considerable space to the history of the town of Lourdes, France, a Catholic shrine famous for the miracles that have allegedly occurred there. "The public relations people who sell Lourdes as a business," says Randi, "claim that there are about 30,000 healings a year, but church authorities deny that figure, cautioning that only about 100 claims have been properly documented since the founding of the shrine, and the church has as of this date accepted only 64 as miracles, from the millions of cures claimed over the years" (20).

Have there been miraculous cures at Lourdes, or anywhere else for that matter? Randi doesn't think so. "I have been willing to accept just *one* case of a miracle cure," he writes, "so that I might say in this book that at least on one occasion a miracle has occurred" (25). But what qualifies as a "miraculous cure"? Randi's criteria are these:

1. The disease must be not normally self-terminating.
2. The recovery must be complete.
3. The recovery must take place in the absence of any medical treatment that might normally be expected to affect the disease.
4. There must be adequate medical opinion that the disease was present before the application of whatever means were used to bring about the miracle.
5. There must be adequate medical opinion that the disease is not present after the application of whatever means were used to bring about the miracle.

Randi insists that he has tried to obtain from all possible sources "direct, examinable evidence that faith-healing occurs" (287). To this point he has failed to obtain a response from any faith healer that satisfies the requirements outlined above.

Randi's outrage is not restricted to claims concerning bodily healing. He is no less determined to expose the financial excesses of those involved in healing ministries and what he believes is the fraudulent use of the United States postal service to raise money. Randi sets his sights particularly on Oral Roberts and Peter Popoff (though W. V. Grant and Leroy Jenkins also come in for criticism). He describes in disturbing detail Roberts's most recent attempts to raise money, a ploy Randi calls religious "extortion." Roberts's claim that God would "take him home" if he did not raise $8 million was soon followed by the announcement that Satan had also tried to take his life. Has it occurred to him, asks Randi, "that he doesn't have many friends in high—or low—places? When God *and* Satan are trying to do you in, there's a message in it somewhere" (65).

The financial empires built by Peter Popoff and W. V. Grant are also subjected to careful scrutiny. The mere fact that such men as these have amassed huge personal fortunes does not rankle Randi. What *is* particularly disturbing to him is that they seem to have done so under false pretenses and at the expense, both financial and emotional, of thousands of devoted followers. Randi explains how mailing campaigns are carefully orchestrated to generate remarkable sums of money. At one time, says Randi, Peter Popoff was receiving an average of $1.25 million a month from mail income *alone*. His conclusion reflects the disdain he feels for such men.

It appears that the easy, foolproof way to get rich in America is to learn about twenty quotations from the Bible, dress in an expensive suit with lots of gaudy jewelry, and rent an auditorium. Tell all the lies you want. Exaggerate your history or invent it entirely. Label all your opponents as "tools of Satan." Answer any and all arguments and objections by quoting scripture. Beg for money, incessantly. Oh. I almost forgot. Ordain yourself as an Anointed Minister of God. Then watch the money roll in. It's tax-free, and you can use it any way you want (73).

Randi's discussion of several prominent faith-healers constitutes the central focus of the book. Following brief chapters on A. A. Allen and Leroy Jenkins, Randi opens fire on men with whom we are more familiar. He begins with W. V. Grant.

Randi's portrait of Grant is not a flattering one. He uncovers several discrepancies in Grant's personal history and documents the various (and, according to Randi, *nefarious*) ways in which Grant has built his religious and financially lucrative empire. Especially disturbing is the evidence Randi has amassed concerning outright deception and trickery in Grant's healing services. For example, people who enter Grant's services fully capable of walking under their own power are placed in wheelchairs provided by Grant's associates. Later they are "healed" of their disability and "miraculously" rise up to walk. Not only do they walk, but Grant has them push *him* in the wheelchair to the obvious delight of the crowd! Grant's methods for healing the "blind" and the "deaf," as well as his ability to lengthen legs, are also subjected to rigorous scrutiny, and found wanting.

Perhaps Randi's most important discovery relates to the way in which Grant obtained his detailed information concerning the people whom he would heal. Grant claims to receive the data directly from God by means of "the word of knowledge," one of the many spiritual gifts mentioned in 1 Corinthians 12 (see chapter 10). In reality, Grant obtained the information well in advance of the healing service. Often his aides would interview the people whom Grant would later "call out" for healing. Some of the information was gleaned from letters Grant received by mail. In any case, he would memorize as much of the personal details as possible, and what he could not remember was committed to crib-sheets carried with him into the service, one of which Randi has obtained and reproduced in the book. Numerous other discoveries Randi has made relating to Grant's personal life are both sensationalistic and salacious. If your curiosity demands satisfaction, I can only recommend that you read the book.

Peter Popoff is Randi's next target. There is extensive documentation of Popoff's questionable methods of fund raising. Randi mentions several items sold by Popoff to his naive followers.

> One such piece was a "Holy Shower Cap." This was a cheap plastic affair that was to be worn by the recipient and then wrapped around some cash or a check and mailed back to Popoff. As such things go, it was a relative failure; it brought in only $100,000 from a single mailing. Some other gimmicks were: holy gloves (throw-away vinyl work gloves), golden prosperity envelopes, special red faith strings, mustard seeds, gold and silver lamé patches, holy ribbons, blessed shoe liners, sanctified handprints, Russian rubles, and red felt hearts. There were also sacred handkerchiefs imbued with the preacher's sweat. Popoff bought 36,000 of these from Synanon, another religious organization, at 25¢ apiece. He tore each into three pieces and represented to the faithful that he had mopped his brow with each scrap he mailed out (140-41).

In addition, the specially "anointed oil" which Popoff would send for an offering of 30 dollars was not, as he claimed, obtained in the Holy Land. It was a mixture of olive oil and Old Spice shaving lotion.

The most damning indictment of Popoff was the revelation that the information about people in the audience he claimed to have received from God was actually being transmitted to him by his wife backstage. One of Randi's assistants discovered that Popoff was wearing a small electronic device in his ear. The radio transmission, on 39.170 megahertz, originated with Elizabeth Popoff who would read him personal data gleaned from interviews conducted prior to the meeting. The results of Randi's exposé of Popoff on national television are recounted in full. When combined with the numerous other scams run by Popoff, it is no wonder that he has virtually disappeared from any form of televised ministry.

Randi also devotes chapters to Oral Roberts and Pat Robertson (although in my opinion Pat Robertson does not belong in the same category with Grant, Popoff, and Roberts; were Robertson not running for the presidency, I doubt that Randi would have said much about him). There isn't much new in this material. These men are perhaps the most visible and best known of TV preachers, and their personal histories are a matter of public record. Of special interest, however, is Randi's persistent appeal to both men that they provide him with at least one authentic case of someone who has been miraculously healed. Randi insists he has diligently sought such evidence. He also insists that neither Roberts nor Robertson has made any response.

Reverend Willard Fuller is also grist for Randi's mill. Fuller calls himself "The Psychic Dentist" and claims to be empowered by God to fill teeth and supply gold crowns to those suffering from dental problems. Says Randi: "I have one simple question regarding Willard Fuller: How is it that he not only wears thick glasses to correct his eyesight, but also has six teeth missing himself, while the rest are badly stained and contain quite ordinary silver fillings? Physician, heal thyself" (212).

There are a dozen or so other faith healers whom Randi discusses and dissects, but there is no need for me to comment on them. The story is much the same with each. What we need to do now is to turn our attention to Randi himself.

Randi's Presuppositions

I must first of all say that I join with James Randi in his anger and dismay at the fraudulent practices of many faith healers. I agree with him that legal action should be taken against those who, for their own financial profit, deliberately and maliciously deceive the public. Freedom of religious expression does not give the shepherd a right to fleece the flock.

But as I read this book, it also became evident to me that I was reading more than an indictment of faith healing. I was reading an indictment of Christianity in general. In fact, I got the distinct impression that as far as Randi is concerned, if the former is fraudulent and discredited, so is the latter. In order to substantiate this we need only examine several of Randi's own beliefs.

Let's begin with his concept of "faith." He first quotes a definition of faith provided by H. L. Mencken: "Faith may be defined briefly as an illogical belief in the occurrence of the improbable." Randi then cites the definitions of faith found in the *International Webster New Encyclopedia Dictionary*: "confidence or trust in a person or thing; . . . belief not substantiated by proof; spiritual acceptance of truth or realities not certified by reason; . . . belief in the doctrines or teachings of a religion" (6). These definitions, says Randi, "should satisfy most persons" (6).

Well, they don't satisfy me. To define faith as "belief not substantiated by proof" is misleading. I have "faith" in the bodily resurrection of Jesus, perhaps the greatest of all miracles. But I am also persuaded that there is overwhelming historical and logical proof that it occurred just as the Bible says that it did. Again, to suggest that the doctrines Christians believe "are not certified by reason" is a caricature. I am persuaded that it is eminently reasonable to have faith in the claims of Christianity. Randi is clearly out of order when he sets faith and reason in opposition to each other.

I suspect that Randi conceives of faith in this way because he wants to portray advocates of faith healing as irrational fools, the sort of people who shut their eyes to all evidence other than that which supports their cherished belief. Undoubtedly some who believe in faith healing are so inclined. But to suggest or even remotely imply that this is the nature of Christian faith *per se* is without warrant.

Randi reveals his concept of Christian faith and his bias against religion as a whole in another statement. "It is a common aspect of all religious groups that they simply do not wish to know the truth, but they are fond of saying that they seek the truth; in some cases, they do seek the truth, but on their terms and with their definitions" (280). Randi then gives three examples of this kind of religious thinking. Two of his examples are instances in which

Roman Catholics have claimed to witness a weeping/bleeding statue or picture of the Virgin Mary. Their persistent belief in these alleged occurrences despite strong evidence to the contrary is what Randi considers typical of the religious mind. His third example is the controversy over the authenticity of the Book of Mormon. The efforts by Mormon officials to suppress objective historical analysis of their most sacred book is again treated as standard fare for all Christians! But it is absurd for Randi to identify this mentality with religious people as a whole, particularly Protestant evangelicals.

Randi's disdain for the supernatural is especially evident when he addresses the subject of demons. While I agree with Randi that many faith healers are misguided in blaming all disease and disaster on the devil, I cannot join him in relegating the demonic to mere superstition. He argues that "only one who has not looked into the state of modern religion can possibly fail to know that the Dark Ages, in many respects, are still with us. To millions and millions of otherwise sensible people, demons, devils, imps, and various other supernatural critters are quite literally real" (52). Such "medieval nonsense" (55), as Randi calls it, is embraced by "all Christians who believe in the Holy Bible" (55).

Surely if one believes in the Bible, one must grant the reality of demonic beings. But the only "medieval nonsense" here is on the part of those whose minds are so closed that they refuse to acknowledge the overwhelming evidence for the inspiration and authority of God's Word.

Science is evidently Randi's sole, sufficient authority for determining what is truth. Yet he has a strange notion of what constitutes scientific thinking. He cites with approval the explanation of scientific reasoning provided by Carlo Lastrucci in his book *The Scientific Approach*. Let me quote him exactly as Randi has quoted him. According to Lastrucci:

> All events have a natural cause. . . . This postulate epitomizes the great historical break of modern science away from fundamentalist religion, on the one hand, and from spiritualism and magic on the other. It implies, in effect, that explanations shall be sought in natural causes or antecedents. . . . It eschews supernatural definitions of phenomena, and rejects

the notion that forces, agents or agencies other than those found in nature operate to influence the cosmos, the earth and its flora and fauna. When a supposedly supernatural or extranatural explanation is offered for a perplexing phenomenon, the scientist assumes that the answer will be found in natural forces or events. And until such time that he can explain the event in natural terms, he rejects the belief that some other order of explanation is necessary. If the history of science proves anything, it proves that the scientist has not yet had his confidence in this belief shaken to date (258).

In all candor, that is one of the most *unscientific* statements I have ever read. Instead of defining true science it offers a defense of philosophical naturalism. To declare that "all events have a natural cause" is itself a statement of faith. It can be made only by someone who has already presupposed that God does not exist or, if he does exist, has nothing to do with the natural order of things. But what scientific observation, law, or experiment has yielded the incontrovertible conclusion that God does not exist?

Lastrucci and Randi say that modern science seeks explanations only in natural causes or antecedents. Why? The only answer is that practitioners of this "science" have already arbitrarily and unscientifically excluded the possibility of other, supernatural causes and antecedents. What we have, then, is Lastrucci's own philosophical beliefs *about* science, not a definition of science. He says that modern science "eschews supernatural definitions of phenomena." But true science is allegedly predisposed toward no particular definition of phenomena, and eschews no explanation of reality except those not warranted by the evidence.

The bottom line for Randi is that if an event can be understood and explained, God didn't do it. Or, to put it in other terms, as our knowledge of physical reality increases, our need for a supernatural being decreases. Unlike the unenlightened and medieval mind of prescientific days, we don't need to appeal to some transcendent Deity to explain natural phenomena. In other words, God is no longer necessary. As man has grown up intellectually, God has become more and more like a distant grandfather, of whom we have warm thoughts and fond memories, but who is practically irrelevant to our experience.

Such reasoning is horribly misinformed. It posits an unwarranted dichotomy between nature and super-nature. Why must one assume that if an event can be explained "naturally," God had nothing to do with it? This presupposes that *if* there is a God, he only acts supernaturally. But God acts through and by means of natural phenomena to accomplish his purposes. So-called "natural law" is nothing more or less than *God's* will imposed on *God's* creation. It is *in* and *by* Christ, says the apostle Paul, that all things hold together (Col. 1:17). In him, again says Paul, "we live and move and exist" (Acts 17:28).

Permit me to repeat something I said earlier in chapter 5. There I insisted that in every case the body's recuperative power is traceable to its Creator. If an aspirin relieves your headache, don't thank the pharmaceutical company. Give thanks to God, for it is he who supplied nature with the ingredients that compose the aspirin and he who created, sustains, and enables the body to respond positively to its medicinal properties. The same may be said for any and all medical cures. All genuine healing, whether miraculous or not, is ultimately the work of God. If we believe that God is Lord over all creation and that every natural, physical, and chemical process is subject to his will, surely whatever healing comes via those means is no less "divine" than those healings we refer to as "miraculous." God is no less deserving of glory and honor when he destroys cancer cells through radiation treatment than when he does it directly, apart from some secondary instrumentality.

Conclusions

What are the results of James Randi's investigation? As I see it, Randi has succeeded in exposing a number of fraudulent faith healers in America. He has reminded us that some people use Christianity as a front for personal aggrandizement and financial gain. He has provided us with concrete illustrations of what our Lord meant when he warned us of "false prophets" who come to us in sheep's clothing but inwardly are ravenous wolves (Matt. 7:15).

And he has proved that in churches across our land there are far too many naive and gullible people who know little about the Bible and even less about human nature. For this we are in Randi's debt. And yes, I do recommend you read his book.

Has Randi proved that divine healing is a baseless superstition? Does the deceptive and sinful subterfuge of a handful of unscrupulous evangelists discredit all ministers of the gospel, or perhaps even the gospel itself? No! God forbid! I think even Randi must admit that to draw any such conclusion is both unscientific and unreasonable.

But there is one last order of business. What are we to make of Randi's persistent request that he be provided with documentation and medical evidence that a miraculous healing has really occurred? Should those who believe they have experienced healing from God refuse to cooperate with Randi simply because he is an unbeliever and a self-confessed "secular humanist"?

On the one hand, the truth need never fear scrutiny. Christians certainly have nothing to hide. If our great and glorious God is healing people today, I can think of no good reason to withhold evidence of it from non-Christians. On the other hand, C. Peter Wagner wisely reminds us that "if people believe that God does not heal today, they will not be able to see divine healing, no matter what quantity of documentation or proof is provided. Convincing a skeptic is a thankless effort."[1]

I am often told that miracles and signs and wonders are needed in our day to convince an unbelieving world of the truth of Christ's claims. Personally, I disagree. The greatest worker of miracles who ever lived, the Lord Jesus Christ, had only a handful of followers at the end of his earthly ministry. Miracles, in and of themselves, are not the answer. I agree with Abraham: "If they do not listen to Moses and the Prophets, neither will they be persuaded if someone rises from the dead" (Luke 16:31). Unbelief is not principally an intellectual problem that can be overcome by more and more facts. It is fundamentally a moral problem, the only solution to which is repentance.

NOTES

Chapter 1: The Healing Phenomenon

1. In one important sense all Christians are "charismatic." All Christians are graciously endowed with at least one spiritual gift, or "charisma." However, I will be using the term in reference to those who both espouse and practice the theological perspective characteristic of the movement that bears the name. By no means is "charismatic" a term of derision or ridicule. I employ it merely as a convenient (even if not always precise) means of identification. Nor do I mean to imply that all charismatics are theologically of one mind. In his excellent book, *A Different Gospel* (Peabody: Hendrickson, 1988), D. R. McConnell insists on distinguishing between the charismatic renewal, which he believes is biblical, and the "Faith" movement (also known as the "Word" or the "Word of Faith" movement), in which he sees heretical and even "cultic" features. Although the distinction McConnell draws is a valid one, I have made no attempt in this study to differentiate between charismatic authors in the way that he suggests. (Among the principal figures in the "Faith" movement, McConnell includes Kenneth Hagin, Kenneth and Gloria Copeland, Frederick Price, Charles Capps, Norvel Hayes, and Robert Tilton, just to mention a few.) Finally, it should also be noted that not all noncharismatics are theologically of the same mind either. Many noncharismatics affirm a cessationist view of the charismata, insisting that miracle gifts as well as signs and wonders ceased in or soon after the first century A.D. Other noncharismatics, such as myself, do not believe the biblical evidence demands a cessationist interpretation. The only gift which I believe the New Testament explicitly restricts to the first century is that of apostleship, narrowly defined.

2. James I. Packer (*Keep in Step With the Spirit* [Old Tappan: Fleming H. Revell, 1984]) has noted that "charismatic preoccupation with experience observably inhibits the long, hard theological and ethical reflection for which the New Testament letters so plainly call. The result often is naiveté and imbalance in handling the biblical revelation" (192).

3. Kenneth E. Hagin, *I Believe in Visions* (Old Tappan: Fleming H. Revell, 1972), 13-14.

4. Norvel Hayes, *How to Live and Not Die* (Tulsa: Harrison House, 1986), 120.

5. Ibid., 107-8.

6. See the discussion of Branham and his influence on contemporary healing ministries in David Edwin Harrell, Jr., *All Things Are Possible: The Healing and Charismatic Revivals in Modern America* (Bloomington: Indiana University Press, 1975), 27-41.

7. Paul Kurtz, "Deceit in the Name of God: What Can Be Done?" *Free Inquiry* 6 (Summer 1986):5.

8. Ibid. Documentation of this and other questionable activities is provided in a series of articles in *Free Inquiry* 6 (Spring 1986) and 6 (Summer 1986). An extensive exposé of these men and their practices has been provided by James Randi in his new book, *The Faith-Healers* (Buffalo: Prometheus, 1987). For my review of Randi's book, see Appendix C.

9. John Wimber and Kevin Springer, *Power Healing* (London: Hodder and Stoughton, 1986), 29.

10. Lewis B. Smedes, ed., *Ministry and the Miraculous: A Case Study at Fuller Theological Seminary* (Pasadena: Fuller Theological Seminary, 1987), 44, 48.

11. Ibid., 48-49. See also the brief but helpful treatment in the editorial, "Miracles Then and Now," *Themelios* 12 (September 1986): 1-4.

12. Colin Brown, *That You May Believe: Miracles and Faith Then and Now* (Grand Rapids: Eerdmans, 1985), 37.

13. Ibid., 64.

14. Packer, *Keep in Step*, 193-94.

15. David Allan Hubbard, *Ministry and the Miraculous*, 11.

16. Packer, *Keep in Step*, 194.

Chapter 2: Two Crucial Texts: Hebrews 13:8 and Isaiah 53:4-5

1. Rodney Clapp, in his article "Faith Healing: A Look at What's Happening" (*Christianity Today*, December 16, 1983), tells the story of the miraculous healing of Barbara Cummiskey. She was also healed of MS after suffering for 15 years with this debilitating disease.

2. Gloria Copeland, *And Jesus Healed Them All* (Ft. Worth: KCP, 1984), 4.

3. See my book *The Grandeur of God: A Theological and Devotional Study of the Divine Attributes* (Grand Rapids: Baker, 1984), 107-16.

4. Quoted in Henry W. Frost, *Miraculous Healing* (Grand Rapids: Zondervan, 1972), 42.

5. Copeland, *And Jesus Healed Them All*, 2.

6. Colin Urquhart, *Receive Your Healing* (London: Hodder and Stoughton, 1986), 38.

7. T. J. McCrossan, *Bodily Healing and the Atonement*, re-ed. Roy Hicks and Kenneth E. Hagin (Tulsa: Faith Library, 1982 [1930]), 12.

8. Kenneth E. Hagin, *Healing Belongs to Us* (Tulsa: Faith Library, 1969), 16.

9. Hugh Jeter, *By His Stripes: A Biblical Study on Divine Healing* (Springfield, Mo.: Gospel Publishing House, 1977), 90.

Chapter 3: Healing and Happiness

1. Francis MacNutt, *Healing* (Toronto: Bantam, 1974), 88.

2. Francis MacNutt, *The Power to Heal* (Notre Dame: Ave Maria Press, 1977), 139.

3. Kenneth E. Hagin, *Seven Things You Should Know About Divine Healing* (Tulsa: Faith Library, 1979), 26.

Chapter 4: Healing, Faith, and the Will of God

1. F. F. Bosworth, *Christ the Healer* (Old Tappan: Fleming H. Revell, 1973), 80.

2. Gloria Copeland, *God's Will for Your Healing* (Ft. Worth: Kenneth Copeland Ministries, 1972), 3.

3. Ibid., 9. Kenneth Hagin, in his booklet *Seven Things You Should Know About Divine Healing* (Tulsa: Faith Library, 1983), says much the same thing: "I am fully convinced—I would die saying it so—that it is the plan of Our Father God, in His great love and in His great mercy, that no believer should ever be sick; that every believer should live his full lifespan down here on this earth; and that every believer should finally just fall asleep in Jesus" (21).

4. Colin Urquhart, *Receive Your Healing* (London: Hodder and Stoughton, 1986), 49.

5. Gloria Copeland, *And Jesus Healed Them All* (Ft. Worth: KCP, 1984), 3.

6. Ibid.

7. Urquhart, *Receive Your Healing*, 89.

8. Copeland, *And Jesus Healed Them All*, 11.

9. Urquhart, *Receive Your Healing*, 18.

10. See Garry Friesen with J. Robin Maxson, *Decision Making and the Will of God: A Biblical Alternative to the Traditional View* (Portland: Multnomah Press, 1980).

11. Dave Hunt and T. A. McMahon, *The Seduction of Christianity: Spiritual Discernment in the Last Days* (Eugene: Harvest House, 1985), 26. A good example of what Hunt has in mind is found in the following statement by Norvel Hayes. In his book *How to Live and Not Die* (Tulsa: Harrison House, 1986), Hayes says that whatever you *say* Jesus is, that is what he must be: "If you confess Jesus as your healer, He becomes that to you. If you confess Him as your miracle worker, He becomes that to you. He is to you, *right now*, what you confess Him to be" (106).

12. Joni Eareckson Tada and Steve Estes, *A Step Further* (Grand Rapids: Zondervan, 1978), 129.

13. Ibid., 130.

14. Ibid., 131.

15. J. I. Packer in the foreword to David Watson, *Fear No Evil: One Man Deals With Terminal Illness* (Wheaton: Harold Shaw, 1984), 7.

Chapter 5: Is There a Doctor in the House?

1. Rodney Clapp, "Faith Healing: A Look at What's Happening," *Christianity Today*, December 16, 1983, 14.

2. Jim Hayes as told to Angela Kiesling, "The Doctor Who Was Healed," *Charisma*, September 1986, 21.

3. The "Healing Explosion" is a ministry of Charles and Francis Hunter, described by one author as "the Ozzie and Harriet of faith healing." Crowds of up to ten thousand are attending these meetings, at which the Hunters not only pray for and lay hands on the sick but also train others to do so as well. A brief description of their ministry is found in Steven Lawson's article, "Hunters' Healing Meetings Explosive," *Charisma*, October 1986, 76-77.

4. Bruce Barron, *The Health and Wealth Gospel* (Downers Grove: Inter-Varsity Press, 1987), 42.

5. Ibid.

6. David Edwin Harrel, *All Things Are Possible: The Healing and Charismatic Revivals in Modern America* (Bloomington: Indiana University Press, 1975), 62.

7. The details have been ably set forth by Barron in his book, *The Health and Wealth Gospel*, 14-34.

8. Hobart Freeman, *Faith for Healing* (Warsaw, Ind.: Faith, n.d.), 10.

9. Barron, *The Health and Wealth Gospel*, 26.

10. Ibid., 22.

11. "Oklahoma death puts parents' faith on trial," *The Dallas Morning News*, September 9, 1984, 52A.

12. For a defense of this approach, see Francis MacNutt, *Healing* (Toronto: Bantam, 1974), 240.

13. Barron, *The Health and Wealth Gospel*, 84.

14. Ibid., 85.

15. Hugh Jeter, *By His Stripes: A Biblical Study on Divine Healing* (Springfield, Mo.: Gospel Publishing House, 1977), 133.

16. John Wimber, *Power Healing* (London: Hodder and Stoughton, 1986), 212.

17. Ibid., 212-13.

18. Blaine Cook, "Taking Healing Home," *Charisma*, September 1986, 34.

19. Colin Urquhart, *Receive Your Healing* (London: Hodder and Stoughton, 1986), 92.

20. Ibid., 93.

21. Paul Brand with Philip Yancey, "A Surgeon's View of Divine Healing," *Christianity Today*, November 25, 1983, 16.

22. Ibid.

Chapter 6: Satan, Sin, and Suffering

1. See the Addendum, "Joni on Job and His God."

2. Norvel Hayes, *How to Live and Not Die* (Tulsa: Harrison House, 1986), 9.

3. Francis I. Anderson, *Job: An Introduction and Commentary* (Downer's Grove: Inter-Varsity Press, 1976), 88.

4. Frederick K. Price, *Is Healing for All?* (Tulsa: Harrison House, 1976), 10.

5. Ibid.

6. Joni Eareckson Tada and Steve Estes, *A Step Further* (Grand Rapids: Zondervan, 1978), 36-37.

Chapter 7: Why Did Jesus Heal the Sick?

1. Lewis B. Smedes, *Ministry and the Miraculous: A Case Study at Fuller Theological Seminary* (Pasadena: Fuller Theological Seminary, 1987), 27.

2. D. A. Carson, *Showing the Spirit* (Grand Rapids: Baker, 1987), 156.

3. Ibid., 151.

4. Ibid., 154.

5. Ibid., 155.

6. Michael Harper, *The Healings of Jesus* (Downers Grove: Inter-Varsity Press, 1986), 63.

Chapter 8: How Did Jesus Heal the Sick?

1. For an explanation of the distinction between organic and functional disorders, see William A. Nolen, *Healing: A Doctor in Search of a Miracle* (New York: Random House, 1974), 259-69; and John Wimber, *Power Healing* (London: Hodder and Stoughton, 1986), 141-48.

2. Donald A. Carson, *Matthew*, The Expositor's Bible Commentary (Grand Rapids: Zondervan, 1984), 8:336.
3. Francis MacNutt, *The Power to Heal* (Notre Dame: Ave Maria Press, 1977), 27.
4. Ibid., 29.
5. Ibid., 45.
6. Marilyn Hickey in *Charisma* magazine, May 1987, 13.
7. Wimber, *Power Healing*, 157.
8. Ibid., 158. A similar approach is taken by Jim Glennon, *Your Healing Is Within You* (Plainfield, N.J.: Logos International, 1980), 170-72.
9. Michael Harper, *The Healings of Jesus* (Downers Grove: Inter-Varsity Press, 1986), 108.
10. John Calvin, *A Harmony of the Gospels: Matthew, Mark and Luke*, trans. T. H. L. Parker (Grand Rapids: Eerdmans, 1972), 2:182.
11. Carson, *Matthew*, 8:265.
12. Donald A. Carson, *The Farewell Discourse and Final Prayer of Jesus: An Exposition of John 14-17* (Grand Rapids: Baker, 1980), 42.

Chapter 9: Healing in the Book of Acts
1. See the article by P. W. Van Der Horst, "Peter's Shadow: The Religio-Historical Background of Acts v. 15," *New Testament Studies* 23 (January 1977):204-12.
2. John Wimber, *Power Evangelism* (San Francisco: Harper and Row, 1986), 98. C. Peter Wagner essentially agrees with the view taken by Wimber. See his *How to Have a Healing Ministry Without Making Your Church Sick!* (Ventura: Regal, 1988).
3. T. J. McCrossan, *Bodily Healing and the Atonement*, re-ed. Roy Hicks and Kenneth E. Hagin (Tulsa: Faith Library, 1982 [1930]), 35.
4. Ibid., 3, emphasis mine.
5. Kenneth E. Hagin, *Seven Things You Should Know About Divine Healing* (Tulsa: Faith Library, 1979), 13.
6. Richard N. Longenecker, *The Acts of the Apostles*, The Expositor's Bible Commentary (Grand Rapids: Zondervan, 1981), 9:492.

Chapter 10: Healing in the Epistles
1. See Hugh Jeter, *By His Stripes: A Biblical Study on Divine Healing* (Springfield, Mo.: Gospel Publishing House, 1977), 152-53.
2. Ibid., 152.
3. John Wimber, *Power Healing* (London: Hodder and Stoughton, 1986), 204.
4. John Wimber, *Power Evangelism* (San Francisco: Harper and Row, 1986), 32. It would appear that what Wimber calls the "word of knowledge" Wayne Grudem calls the gift of "prophecy." See Grudem's book, *The Gift of Prophecy in the New Testament and Today* (Westchester: Crossway, 1988).
5. Robert Tilton, pastor of Word of Faith in Dallas, Texas, has given a new twist to the word of knowledge. He now claims that God imparts knowledge to him of people who should donate money to his ministry. The remarkable thing is that Tilton insists God even specifies the exact dollar amount that the individual is to give!
6. Michael Harper, *The Healings of Jesus* (Downers Grove: Inter-Varsity Press, 1986, 27.

164   NOTES

7. Ibid., 49.
8. Wimber, *Power Evangelism*, 62.
9. Wimber, *Power Healing*, 192. Wimber also believes that closely related to the word of knowledge is the gift of discerning spirits, which he says "is especially important for knowing how to pray accurately for a person's healing" (ibid., 204).
10. Harper, *The Healings of Jesus*, 27.
11. Ralph P. Martin, *The Spirit and the Congregation: Studies in 1 Corinthians 12-15* (Grand Rapids: Eerdmans, 1984), 13.
12. James D. G. Dunn, *Jesus and the Spirit: A Study of the Religious and Charismatic Experience of Jesus and the First Christians as Reflected in the New Testament* (Philadelphia: Westminster Press, 1975), 217.
13. Ibid.
14. Gordon D. Fee, *The First Epistle to the Corinthians* (Grand Rapids: Eerdmans, 1987), 591.
15. Martin, *The Spirit and the Congregation*, 13.
16. Dunn, *Jesus and the Spirit*, 220.
17. Fee, *The First Epistle to the Corinthians*, 593.
18. Richard M. Sipley, *Understanding Divine Healing* (Wheaton, Victor, 1986), 135.
19. Gerald F. Hawthorne, *Philippians*, Word Biblical Commentary (Waco: Word, 1983), 120.
20. Sipley, *Understanding Divine Healing*, 69; and Jeter, *By His Stripes*, 106.
21. J. N. D. Kelly, *A Commentary on the Pastoral Epistles* (London: Adam and Charles Black, 1963), 129.
22. Jeter, *By His Stripes*, 131.
23. See Raymond E. Brown, "Appendix V: General Observations on Epistolary Format" in *The Epistles of John*, The Anchor Bible (Garden City: Doubleday and Company, 1982, 788-95; and Gordon Fee and Douglas Stuart, *How to Read the Bible for All It's Worth* (Grand Rapids: Zondervan, 1982), 44-46.
24. Fee and Stuart, *How to Read the Bible*, 44.
25. I. Howard Marshall, *The Epistles of John* (Grand Rapids: Eerdmans, 1978), 83.

Chapter 11: Paul's Thorn in the Flesh
1. John Calvin, *The Second Epistle of Paul the Apostle to the Corinthians and the Epistles to Timothy, Titus and Philemon*, trans. T. A. Small (Grand Rapids: Eerdmans, 1973), 160.
2. Ralph P. Martin, *2 Corinthians*, Word Biblical Commentary (Waco: Word, 1986), 412. One among many good examples of the "divine passive" is found in Matt. 7:2.
3. Victor Paul Furnish, *II Corinthians*, The Anchor Bible (Garden City: Doubleday and Company, 1984), 528.
4. Martin, *2 Corinthians*, 412.
5. Perhaps *epitithēmi*, "lay upon" (Luke 10:30; 23:26; Acts 16:23), or *ballō*, "cast" (Rev. 2:24), or *epiballō*, "put on" (1 Cor. 7:35) would be more appropriate to describe Satanic action. See Martin, *2 Corinthians*, 412.
6. Donald A. Carson, *From Triumphalism to Maturity: An Exposition of 2 Corinthians 10-13* (Grand Rapids: Baker, 1984), 144.

7. Joni Eareckson Tada and Steve Estes, *A Step Further* (Grand Rapids: Zondervan, 1978), 145-46.

8. Charles Capps (*Paul's Thorn in the Flesh* [Dallas: Word of Faith, 1983]) offers a totally fanciful interpretation of the purpose of Paul's thorn in the flesh. According to Capps, when Paul says "to keep me from exalting myself," he is referring "to the fact that if it had not been for the messenger of Satan assigned against Paul to stir up trouble, to cause him problems everywhere he preached, Paul's revelations would have been exalted till they would have influenced the whole nation. But he was not able to preach them freely, for Satan hindered him on every hand" (14). In the first place, it was *Paul* who was inclined to self-exaltation, not his "revelations." Perhaps what Capps means is that Paul would himself have been exalted above measure in the sense that everyone would have listened to his gospel and would have accepted it as true, had not Satan prevented it from happening. But this is in conflict with the fact that this "revelation" Paul received was never intended to be proclaimed to others. It was given to him in "inexpressible words, which a man is not permitted to speak" (12:4). It would seem that in his desperate attempt to evade the force of this passage, Capps has turned it upside down. In other words, Capps argues that Paul's thorn in the flesh was not a good thing to keep him from doing a bad thing, but a bad thing to keep him from doing a good thing!

9. R. V. G. Tasker, *The Second Epistle of Paul to the Corinthians* (Grand Rapids: Eerdmans, 1977), 176.

10. This is based on the assumption that F. F. Bruce is correct in dating Paul's conversion in approximately A.D. 33. See *Paul: Apostle of the Heart Set Free* (Grand Rapids: Eerdmans, 1977), 475.

11. Martin, *2 Corinthians*, 415.

12. Calvin, *The Second Epistle of Paul the Apostle to the Corinthians*, 159.

13. James I. Packer, "Poor Health May Be the Best Remedy," *Christianity Today*, May 21, 1982, 15.

14. Charles Hodge, *An Exposition of the Second Epistle to the Corinthians* (Grand Rapids: Eerdmans, 1970), 286.

15. Philip Edgcumbe Hughes, *Paul's Second Epistle to the Corinthians* (Grand Rapids: Eerdmans, 1962), 451.

16. Tasker, *The Second Epistle of Paul to the Corinthians*, 179.

Chapter 12: Anointing With Oil and the Prayer of Faith

1. Daniel R. Hayden, "Calling the Elders to Pray," *Bibliotheca Sacra* 138 (July-September 1981):263.

2. Douglas J. Moo, *The Letter of James* (Grand Rapids: Eerdmans, 1985), 184.

3. See Moo's discussion of these two words, ibid., 179-81.

4. Ibid., 180-81.

5. D. Edmond Hiebert, *The Epistle of James: Tests of a Living Faith* (Chicago: Moody Press, 1979), 322. Although I agree with Hiebert's interpretation, it should not be based on the presence or absence of the Greek definite article.

6. Moo, *The Letter of James*, 182.

7. Ibid., 186-87.

8. R. V. G. Tasker, *The General Epistle of James* (Grand Rapids: Eerdmans, 1977), 133.

Chapter 13: "Why You, Lord?" Or, Suffering and God's Providence
1. John Calvin, *Institutes of the Christian Religion*, ed. John T. McNeill, (Philadelphia: Westminster Press, 1975), I:xvii.1.

Chapter 14: "Why Me, Lord?" Or, Suffering and God's Purpose
1. Joni Eareckson Tada and Steve Estes, *A Step Further* (Grand Rapids: Zondervan, 1978), 12.
2. David Watson, *Fear No Evil: One Man Deals With Terminal Illness* (Wheaton: Harold Shaw, 1984), 119.
3. Tada and Estes, *A Step Further*, 17.
4. Charles Colson, "My Cancer and the Good Health Gospel," *Christianity Today*, April 3, 1987, 56.
5. C. S. Lewis, *The Problem of Pain* (New York: Macmillan, 1962), 93.
6. Tada and Estes, *A Step Further*, 94-95.
7. Ibid., 161.
8. Watson, *Fear No Evil*, 135.
9. Francis MacNutt, *Healing* (Toronto: Bantam Books, 1974), 66. This same distinction is made by Ken Blue in his book *Authority to Heal* (Downers Grove: Inter-Varsity Press, 1987), 27-30.

Epilogue
1. Adapted from the account provided by Emanuel Stickelberger in his book, *Calvin*, trans. David Georg Gelzer (London: James Clarke and Co., 1959), 46-49.
2. See, for example, *John Calvin: His Influence in the Western World*, ed. W. Stanford Reid (Grand Rapids: Zondervan, 1982).

Appendix A: The Defeat of the Devil
1. See Peter T. O'Brien, "Principalities and Powers: Opponents of the Church" in *Biblical Interpretation and the Church: The Problem of Contextualization*, ed. D. A. Carson (Nashville: Thomas Nelson, 1984), 110-50.
2. J. B. Lightfoot, *Saint Paul's Epistles to the Colossians and to Philemon* (Grand Rapids: Zondervan, 1976 [1879]), 190.

Appendix B: Was Jesus Ever Sick?
1. Colin Urquhart, *Receive Your Healing* (London: Hodder and Stoughton, 1986), 21. See also Francis MacNutt, *Healing* (Toronto: Bantam, 1974), 66-67.
2. Some of this discussion has been taken from my book, *Reaching God's Ear* (Wheaton: Tyndale House, 1988).

Appendix C: A Review of James Randi's The Faith-Healers
1. C. Peter Wagner, *How to Have a Healing Ministry Without Making Your Church Sick!* (Ventura: Regal, 1988), 144.

BIBLIOGRAPHY

Barnhart, Joseph E. "On the Relative Sincerity of Faith Healers." *Free Inquiry* 6 (Spring 1986):24-29.

Barron, Bruce. *The Health and Wealth Gospel.* Downers Grove: Inter-Varsity Press, 1987.

Baxter, J. Sidlow. *Divine Healing of the Body.* Grand Rapids: Zondervan, 1979.

Benn, Wallace, and Burkill, Mark. "A Theological and Pastoral Critique of the Teaching of John Wimber." *Churchman* 101 (1987):101-13.

Blue, Ken. *Authority to Heal.* Downers Grove: Inter-Varsity Press, 1987.

Bosworth, F. F. *Christ the Healer.* Old Tappan: Fleming H. Revell, 1973.

Brand, Paul, with Yancey, Philip. "A Surgeon's View of Divine Healing." *Christianity Today,* November 25, 1983, 14-21.

Brown, Colin. *That You May Believe: Miracles and Faith Then and Now.* Grand Rapids: Eerdmans, 1985.

Capps, Charles. *Paul's Thorn in the Flesh.* Dallas: Word of Faith, 1983.

Carson, D. A. *Showing the Spirit: A Theological Exposition of 1 Corinthians 12-14.* Grand Rapids: Baker, 1987.

Clapp, Rodney. "Faith Healing: A Look at What's Happening." *Christianity Today,* December 16, 1983, 12-17.

Colson, Charles. "My Cancer and the Good Health Gospel." *Christianity Today,* April 3, 1987, 56.

Copeland, Gloria. *And Jesus Healed Them All.* Ft. Worth: KCP, 1984.

————. *God's Will for Your Healing*. Ft. Worth: Kenneth Copeland Ministries, 1972.

Fee, Gordon D. *The Disease of the Health and Wealth Gospels*. Costa Mesa, Calif.: The Word for Today, 1979.

Fisk, Samuel. *Divine Healing Under the Searchlight*. Schaumburg, Ill.: Regular Baptist Press, 1978.

Frost, Henry W. *Miraculous Healing*. Grand Rapids: Zondervan, 1972.

Gardner, Rex. *Healing Miracles: A Doctor Investigates*. Darton, Longman, and Todd, 1986.

Geisler, Norman. *Signs and Wonders*. Wheaton: Tyndale House, 1988.

Glennon, Jim. *Your Healing Is Within You*. Plainfield, N.J.: Logos International, 1980.

Hagin, Kenneth E. *Healing Belongs to Us*. Tulsa: Faith Library, 1969.

————. *The Key to Scriptural Healing*. Tulsa: Faith Library, 1983.

————. *Seven Things You Should Know About Divine Healing*. Tulsa: Faith Library, 1979.

Harper, Michael. *The Healings of Jesus*. Downers Grove: Inter-Varsity Press, 1986.

Harrel, David Edwin. *All Things Are Possible: The Healing and Charismatic Revivals in Modern America*. Bloomington: Indiana University Press, 1975.

Hayes, Norvel. *How to Live and Not Die*. Tulsa: Harrison House, 1986.

Jeter, Hugh. *By His Stripes: A Biblical Study on Divine Healing*. Springfield, Mo.: Gospel Publishing House, 1977.

Kee, Howard C. *Medicine, Miracle, and Magic in New Testament Times*. Cambridge: Cambridge University Press, 1986.

Kelsey, Morton T. *Healing and Christianity: In Ancient Thought and Modern Times*. New York: Harper and Row, 1973.

Kreeft, Peter. *Making Sense Out of Suffering*. Ann Arbor: Servant, 1986.

Kurtz, Paul. "Does Faith-Healing Work?" *Free Inquiry* 6 (Spring 1986):30-36.

———. "Pat Robertson and the '700 Club.'" *Free Inquiry* 6 (Spring 1986):34.

———. "W. V. Grant's Faith-Healing Act Revisited." *Free Inquiry* 6 (Summer 1986):12-13.

Lane, Anthony. "Editorial: Miracles Then and Now." *Themelios* 12 (September 1986):1-4.

Lawrence, Roy. *Christian Healing Rediscovered: A Guide to Spiritual, Mental, Physical Wholeness.* Downers Grove: Inter-Varsity Press, 1980.

Lewis, C. S. *Miracles.* New York: Macmillan, 1978 (1947).

———. *The Problem of Pain.* New York: Macmillan, 1962.

McConnell, D. R. *A Different Gospel: A Historical and Biblical Analysis of the Modern Faith Movement.* Peabody: Hendrickson, 1988.

McCrossan, T. J. *Bodily Healing and the Atonement.* Re-ed. Roy Hicks and Kenneth E. Hagin. Tulsa: Faith Library, 1982 [1930].

McMahon, William E., and Griffis, James B. "Further Reflections on Ernest Angley." *Free Inquiry* 6 (Summer 1986):15-17.

MacNutt, Francis. *Healing.* Toronto: Bantam, 1974.

———. *The Power to Heal.* Notre Dame: Ave Maria Press, 1977.

Mayhue, Richard. *Divine Healing Today.* Chicago: Moody Press, 1983.

Nolen, William A. *Healing: A Doctor in Search of a Miracle.* New York: Random House, 1974.

Osborn, T. L. *Healing the Sick.* Tulsa: Harrison House, 1959.

Packer, James I. *Keep in Step With the Spirit.* Old Tappan: Fleming H. Revell, 1984.

———. "Poor Health May Be the Best Remedy." *Christianity Today,* May 21, 1982, 14-26.

Price, Frederick K. *Is Healing for All?* Tulsa: Harrison House, 1976.

Randi, James. " 'Be Healed in the Name of God!' An Exposé of the Reverend W. V. Grant." *Free Inquiry* 6 (Spring 1986):8-19.

————. "Peter Popoff Reaches Heaven via 39.17 Megahertz." *Free Inquiry* 6 (Summer 1986):6-7.

————. "W. V. Grant's 'Leg-Stretching Trick.'" *Free Inquiry* 6 (Spring 1986):16.

Reisser, Paul C., Reisser, Teri K., and Weldon, John. *The Holistic Healers: A Christian Perspective on New-Age Health Care.* Downers Grove: Inter-Varsity Press, 1983.

Schafersman, Steven. "Peter Popoff: Miracle Worker or Scam Artist?" *Free Inquiry* 6 (Summer 1986):8-9.

Seybold, Klaus and Mueller, Ulrich B. *Sickness and Healing.* Nashville: Abingdon, 1981.

Signs and Wonders Today. Compiled by the editors of *Christian Life Magazine.* Wheaton: Christian Life Magazine, 1983.

Simson, Eve. *The Faith-Healers: Deliverance Evangelism in North America.* St. Louis: Concordia, 1977.

Singer, Philip. "Grant's 'Miracles': A Follow-up." *Free Inquiry* 6 (Spring 1986):22-23.

————. "A Medical Anthropologist's View of American Shamans." *Free Inquiry* 6 (Spring 1986):20-23.

Sipley, Richard M. *Understanding Divine Healing.* Wheaton: Victor, 1986.

Skinner, R. David. "Is Healing in the Atonement? Or, The Question of Faith-Healing." *Mid-America Theological Journal* 9 (Fall 1985):31-47.

Smedes, Lewis B., ed. *Ministry and the Miraculous: A Case Study at Fuller Theological Seminary.* Pasadena: Fuller Theological Seminary, 1987.

Springer, Kevin, ed. *Power Encounters.* San Francisco: Harper and Row, 1988.

Sproul, R. C. "Buy Now, Pay Later Christianity." *Eternity,* January 1987, 64.

Stafford, Tim. "Testing the Wine From John Wimber's Vineyard." *Christianity Today,* August 8, 1986, 17-22.

Steiner, Robert A. "Behind the Scenes With Peter Popoff." *Free Inquiry* 6 (Summer 1986):10-11.

Tada, Joni Eareckson. *A Step Further.* Grand Rapids: Zondervan, 1978.

Urquhart, Colin. *Receive Your Healing.* London: Hodder and Stoughton, 1986.

Vaux, Kenneth L. *Health and Medicine in the Reformed Tradition: Promise, Providence, and Care.* New York: Crossroad, 1984.

Wacker, Grant. "Wimber and Wonders—What About Miracles Today?" *Reformed Journal* (April 1987):16-19.

Wagner, C. Peter. *How to Have a Healing Ministry Without Making Your Church Sick!* Ventura: Regal, 1988.

————. *The Third Wave of the Holy Spirit: Encountering the Power of Signs and Wonders Today.* Ann Arbor: Servant, 1988.

Watson, David. *Fear No Evil: One Man Deals With Terminal Illness.* Wheaton: Harold Shaw, 1984.

White, John. *When the Spirit Comes With Power: Signs and Wonders Among God's People.* Downers Grove: Inter-Varsity Press, 1988.

Wilkinson, John. *Health and Healing: Studies in New Testament Principles and Practice.* Handsel Press, 1980.

Wimber, John. *Power Evangelism.* San Francisco: Harper and Row, 1986.

————. *Power Healing.* London: Hodder and Stoughton, 1986.

INDEX OF SCRIPTURE

176

INDEX OF PROPER NAMES